8/12/17

To : Ruth G.

From my new ?

HEART ATTACK

to yours

May all your heart beats count!!

M Lopez MD

8/12/17

HEART ATTACK

Truth · Tragedy · Triumph

William A. Cooper,
MD, MBA, FACS, FACC

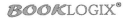
BOOKLOGIX®
Alpharetta, GA

This book is not intended as a substitute for the medical advice of physicians. The reader should consult a physician regularly in any matters relating to his/her health, particularly with respect to any symptoms or illness that may require diagnosis or medical attention.

This ISBN is the property of BookLogix for the express purpose of sales and distribution of this title. The content of this book is the property of the copyright holder only. BookLogix does not hold any ownership of the content of this book and is not liable in any way for the materials contained within. The views and opinions expressed in this book are the property of the Author/Copyright holder, and do not necessarily reflect those of BookLogix.

Copyright © 2016 by Dr. William Cooper

All rights reserved. No part of this book may be reproduced or transmitted in any form or by any means, electronic or mechanical, including photocopying, recording, or any information storage and retrieval system, without permission in writing from the publisher. For more information, address BookLogix, c/o Permissions Department, 1264 Old Alpharetta Rd., Alpharetta, GA 30005.

Cover design by Jacob Mason
Contact: abstractgrafics@msn.com

ISBN: 978-1-61005-730-1
Library of Congress Control Number: 2016911700

10 9 8 7 6 5 4 3 2   0 9 2 1 1 6

Printed in the United States of America

∞This paper meets the requirements of ANSI/NISO Z39.48-1992 (Permanence of Paper)

To my departed family: mother, Arthur Louise; sisters, Vicki, Leslie Nicole, and Janice; and brothers, Alvin and Alex Jr.

CONTENTS

PREFACE

Heart Attack, unlike many books of its kind, takes you on a journey discussing heart disease through the lives of those who have suffered at the hands of this dreadful condition. Beginning with the author's own devastating family history, *Heart Attack* reminds us that we are all connected not just by the physical attributes and risk factors associated with heart attacks, but also emotionally and spiritually. Many of the characters in this book suffered real heart attacks, and others, although perhaps not "heart attacks" of the purest kind, suffered as well.

According to the World Health Organization, each year heart disease accounts for greater than 17 million deaths worldwide [1]. The vast majority, over 7 million, of these deaths involve some form of the loosely applied term "heart attack." By comparison, according to the Centers for Disease Control and Prevention (CDC), over 600,000 Americans die of heart disease each year, which accounts for approximately 25 percent of all deaths for both men and women [2, 3].

This is the way most books on the subject of heart disease begin, with facts and statistics. *Heart Attack* breaks down the statistical barriers to analyze the impact of heart disease on individuals and humanity. Perhaps this realization will empower and motivate the reader to understand this disease and its prevention on a much deeper level.

AMERICA'S HEART DISEASE BURDEN

America's Heart Disease Burden—
Heart Disease Is Not Number One?

Yes, I know you might be thinking—has Dr. Cooper lost his mind? He's a heart doctor, why would he say that? Of course heart disease deaths outpace all other major illness categories combined. Does it? Yes, it does, at least from the perspective lens through which we view it.

One of my objectives when I speak and write on this subject is to change perspectives on how we might view some of the laissez-faire facts, figures, and slogans we hear from various sources on a daily basis. I think we have a tendency to become "comfortable" with these dogmatic (in some ways) issues. We are quite prolific at measuring the output or outcome of a disease process or procedure and reporting it as "the problem."

Contrarily, we tend to gloss over the inputs, the triggers, or the risks that contribute to the development of a particular condition. Why? Because to do so would lead us down the seemingly difficult path of cause, effect, and prevention. Thus we begin to talk prevention and invariably, we have to discuss lifestyles and lifestyle choices, including how we eat, whether we smoke, drink in excess, or get the recommended daily exercise needed to sustain wellness.

According to the Centers for Disease Control and Prevention (CDC), we have a long way to go to get to an ideal level of health and wellness. However, doing so would relieve us (individuals and the health-care system) of a major burden.

Here are some sobering facts:

- We don't get enough exercise. Only 50 percent of us get the recommended daily dose [4]. Remember, its thirty minutes five to six days a week with a goal to achieve your recommended target heart rate. For those who "don't have time," then double the numbers because you will need it in the long run. As far as time is concerned, let me change your perspective again. The recommendation adds up to 1.8 percent; that's three of the 168 hours available in a week. Get busy!

- The risk factor burden is too high. Half of Americans have at least one major risk factor for heart attack and stroke including: high blood pressure, high cholesterol, overweight or obese, or cigarette smoking [2]. Ninety percent of us consume ten times the recommended daily intake of sodium which contributes to high blood pressure [5].

- Dare I mention nutrition? We are barely scratching the surface on this problem. Even worse, our children and adolescents eat horribly. You don't need numbers on this one. All those sexy lattes and frappuccinos are loaded with just about everything you don't need.

- And all of this is costing you money. Health is wealth; without it, it is nearly impossible to achieve financial goals and security. On the contrary, you may not necessarily achieve health by becoming wealthy, as wealth tends to lead to overconsumption. Balance the scale, but I would put my "money" on health first which gives you a much better chance to achieve wealth [5].
  - 90 percent of all health-care expenditures are spent on treating chronic conditions
  - 300 billion on heart disease
  - 250 billion on diabetes
  - 290 billion on smoking-related illnesses
  - 300 billion lost productivity due to chronic disease

Okay, are you with me now? Yes, heart disease is a major "killer" in this country and around the world. And yes, we should continue to focus on efforts to reduce the burden of heart disease on our society through clinical practice, research, and educating the community at large. We won't and shouldn't give up the fight.

Would the real killers please stand up?

TESTIMONIAL
BY JOHN PALMER

I experienced sharp pains in my left and right arm lasting a few seconds on occasion. The pain was centralized from my wrist to elbow area. I didn't have a clue what was causing these pains, but I figured it could not be heart-related because it occurred in both arms. I thought it was associated with working out with weights or swinging a golf club or any number of exercises I did with my trainer.

These episodes occurred once or twice a day, and initially the pain was attention-grabbing but not debilitating. I hesitated in telling my wife, Vicki, because I thought they would eventually go away. Yet through these experiences, I was becoming more and more concerned.

Over the next several days, the pain seemed to become a little sharper. I continued to reason irrationally that it was related to exercise, and I added a new theory. I have been an asthmatic most of my life. As I grew older, asthma attacks happened with less frequency. However, I added asthma to my misdiagnosis. Each time it happened the pain grew worse. It became more intense, approaching debilitating.

On a Saturday morning I had a major episode, and this one was life changing. My wife was preparing to pull out of the garage on her way to a meeting. I had another attack that was so painful, I dropped to my knees and placed my forehead into the carpet with my arms around my back, hands clasped. The pain was excruciating.

This lasted a few seconds. Once the pain subsided, I got on my feet and made a beeline to the garage to catch my wife.

She was backing out of the garage as I opened the door with tears streaming down my face. I screamed, "Stop!" and waved in a flagging motion to make certain she saw me. She came back into the garage a few feet before she turned the ignition off and got out of the car with an "oh my God" look as she screamed, "What's wrong?"

I desperately uttered something like, "I don't know what's wrong! I have terrible pains in both arms. Please take me to a hospital now!" She could see I was sweating, in pain, and scared to death. She went into action assisting me into the car, pulling the seat belt over and around me, then getting a bottle of water. She raced to the hospital while asking me questions about what I was feeling and how long I had been feeling these symptoms. She assured me that everything would be okay and that we would be at the hospital soon.

We arrived at the emergency room, where they took us to an exam room and began asking questions. I told them about the arm pains and that I thought it was an asthma attack. They ruled out asthma and gave me an EKG. As we waited for the results, we overheard the doctor on the phone using words like "radical abnormalities." I asked Vicki if they were talking about me and she said they couldn't be. I was slim and fit. But quietly, Vicki called her administrative assistant, Wanda, and asked her to find Chris Leggett, a close family friend and renowned interventional cardiologist. Meanwhile the cardiology consult in the ER came in and said they would admit me and perform a stress test with dye on Monday.

Dr. Chris Leggett was in his barber's chair getting a haircut when the page from an unknown number came through. He returned the call and Wanda explained the circumstances and asked him to call Vicki. Chris called Vicki immediately. He requested my EKG be faxed to his home. Once getting home and seeing the EKG results and other data, Chris called the cardiac catheterization laboratory at his hospital, St. Joseph, which was across the street from Northside where I was being processed into a room. He ordered an ambulance to pick me up and deliver me to St. Joseph. I said I could walk across the street, and Vicki looked at me with one of those looks of "Did you really say that? You will NOT be walking!"

Chris got into his car and raced to St. Joseph. While on the road, he called his friend and cardiothoracic surgeon who said he was on his way to dinner with his family. Chris asked him to stand by in case he was needed to perform surgery.

The ambulance picked me up and drove across the street to the emergency entrance where I was wheeled into the cath lab and Chris went to work. He was performing the heart catheterization with dye to color and accentuate visibility of what was happening with my heart. He learned that my main artery, a.k.a. "the widow maker," was 99.1 percent blocked. It was so severely blocked the dye was clogging what little remained for blood to flow. I started to feel the extreme pain from my wrist to my elbows again in both arms. I was on the brink of a heart attack and instant death.

Chris ordered three things: to put some quantity of nitroglycerin in my mouth, to insert a balloon which would assist my heart in beating, and, lastly, to charge the paddles to three hundred. The trained doctor in Chris knew that if my heart stopped beating, the defibrillator could not bring me back. Yet Chris, my friend, was fiercely determined to do everything in his power not to have to tell Vicki he had lost me.

The pain subsided and Chris sent word for the cardiothoracic surgeon to rush to the hospital. Once I was stabilized, Chris sat on the side of the gurney, grabbed my hand, and said, "Now let's have prayer."

While I knew something was drastically wrong, I never allowed myself to focus on anything except the fact that I was in extraordinarily competent hands with Chris and that my God had me. Chris left the lab to inform Vicki of my condition. She knew something was wrong because it had taken so long and she saw the cardiothoracic surgeon as he passed her in the lobby. Chris showed her an image of my heart and told her that doctors never saw patients with images like this with a 99.1 percent blockage of the widow-maker artery, because those patients always arrive dead. He then told Vicki he was going to take her into the lab to see me. He made her promise to put on her best "big girl" face, because he really didn't want her to alarm me. When I saw my wife's face, I knew I was at death's door!

I was wheeled to the operating room for what ultimately was a quadruple bypass.

I feel so blessed to have been asked to write the foreword for this amazing book. The numerous lessons contained herein will save thousands of lives. Thanks to the extraordinary skills of Dr. William Cooper and so many incredible cardiologists, sixteen years after that fateful Saturday, I am still here. I work out regularly, eat properly, and do everything within my power to keep my heart healthy.

> "Now faith is the substance of things hoped for . . . the evidence of things not seen."
> -Hebrews 11:1

INTRODUCTION

I believe that the rendering of useful service is the common duty of mankind and that only in the purifying fire of sacrifice is the dross of human selfishness consumed and the greatness of the human soul set free.

-John D. Rockefeller

The First Attacks

As a child growing up in rural southeast Missouri, I would often hear my parents talking about Mr. or Mrs. X or Y having a heart attack and dying as a result. Those times didn't really provoke any meaningful thought in me until much later in my life when I became a physician and heart surgeon. As I think back on those days, two in particular are quite vivid in my memory.

The first occurred when I was about five years old. I was in a pretty bad car accident with Big Mama Ruthie Lumpkin and Big Daddy Orville Lumpkin, who were my babysitters at the time. Of course, we called them Big Mama and Big Daddy in lieu of Mr. and Mrs. Lumpkin.

On this particular day, we were driving along a dirt road near my hometown when a large tractor with a massive cultivator attached to it hit our car. I was standing in the front seat and took a pretty good smack on the windshield. I came close to being one of the statistics that led to the development of child-seat safety laws across the country, and I bear the scars to this day. Big Daddy was driving and Big Mama was sitting in the front passenger seat. I distinctly remember wiping blood from her brow and asking if she was okay. I also remember a thin gentleman in the back seat who was passed out. Not aware at the time, that gentleman was Mama Ruthie's brother. He died that day, my mother later told me, not as a result of the accident, but a heart attack.

Some years later on a hot summer afternoon, my friends Anthony, Bubba (Willie Williams), Draw (Alex Green), and I were running the neighborhood, doing our usual: riding dirt bikes, playing basketball, or building clubhouses, when the all-too-familiar ambulance siren started to blast, breaking the monotony of the day. An ambulance siren in a small town like Hayti, Missouri, was always a big deal, and everyone stopped to see if it was coming their way. Where was it going? Whose house was it today? Who's dying or dead? As the sound became louder and louder, we realized today was our day as the ambulance was turning on Braggadocio Road, heading in our direction.

There was no obstruction to our view as the ambulance headed south toward us on Braggadocio. To the east of the road was a series of single family homes and Joe Kenney's café. To the west and south of the road was an open cotton field, and then the Macks' house where we were playing in the backyard. As the ambulance got closer my friends and I, as well as a number of bystanders along the road, stopped what we were doing and began to track the ambulance. Other cars along the narrow gravel road also stopped to look on.

Finally, it stopped at the last house before the next juke joint. That was the Burnses' house. I recognized the ambulance driver. It was Lawrence Newman, a close family friend and an EMT. He and his assistant got out of the vehicle, unloaded a stretcher, and went inside. The gathering crowd along the road, including my entourage, approached the house to get a closer look. A few minutes passed and then Lawrence and the other EMT emerged from the house with Mr. Burns on the stretcher.

Mrs. Burns, a nurse and EMT herself, was helping attend to Mr. Burns and get the stretcher in the back of the ambulance. She was a tall, well-spoken lady with silver-gray hair. For this victim to be her husband, she was surprisingly calm and composed, as I am sure she had seen this before in her work as a nurse.

This did not look good. Mr. Burns, a dark-skinned man of rather small stature, was ashen in color. He had saliva pouring from his mouth. His body was limp as his arm hung lifelessly over the edge of the stretcher. The EMTs had a bag over his mouth trying to assist with breathing as the other pumped on his chest. They finally got him in the truck and whizzed away.

The crowd quietly dispersed. The boys and I went back to our playground activities. We learned later that evening that Mr. Burns had died of a heart attack.

Throughout my childhood, these scenes repeated themselves often. I can still recall the day my mother got the call that her father had died of a heart attack. Visibly upset and crying, I could only cling to her leg and cry too. I was crying not because I understood what she was feeling. I only knew my mother was upset and I did not like seeing her hurt.

Truth

Since I began writing this book over five years ago, approximately three million people have suffered heart attacks, and over 600,000 of those have died as a result [2].

Remember, "heart disease" does not necessarily imply "heart attack."

But that is not exclusively why I write about heart attacks. Before I go any further with the numbers, I will pause to explain why, at this point in my career, I felt it important to write about such a pervasive issue, one that in some ways is so common that our society has become indifferent to it.

I began my career in medicine in 1986. Nearly thirty years since choosing cardiothoracic surgery as a specialty, I have seen and treated my share of heart attacks. At some point, I began to not only see the heart attack, the x-rays, lab work, and the myriad of tests, but I also began to see people and the human suffering behind those devastating moments.

Often books, reviews, and monographs on this "medical" subject are too sterilized, structured, and focused on numbers. They give generic facts and figures and solutions. The truth is that behind those numbers are human lives affected by this brutal condition. People are afflicted with heart attacks every day, and that suffering should not be buried in statistics. The families and loved ones are also affected, and their experience during these stressful times is no less important.

In Part I of this book, Truth, we will explore the experiences of heart attack victims and the impact on their families. Truth is divided into four chapters, each with a separate focus on family, women, men, and children, respectively. These stories expose a number of fallacies, misfortunes, and inadequacies in our health-care system, our interaction with the system, and our own human nature. The goal is to explore these issues so that the reader may be able to avoid mishap in their own life. Experience is the only true teacher, and it doesn't have to be our own. We can learn much from others.

Tragedy

In Part II, Tragedy, we explore the normal working heart, the risk factors for heart disease, and the conditions that make our hearts sick. The section is presented in a way that is easy to comprehend and put to practical use. Some questions that I commonly come across are addressed in this section.

You might think that the "tragedy" of heart disease is the impact that it has on people as presented in Part I. From my perspective, I believe the tragedy is heart disease itself. This is a condition that most experts believe is largely preventable, and if that is the case, then the tragedy is the fact that it should not be the number-one killer worldwide. Somewhere along the way we have missed something, as heart disease continues to wreak havoc in our lives.

Triumph

In Part III, Triumph, we will explore the successes, failures, and future of prevention and treatment of heart disease. This section is more than the proverbial rhetoric of "just eat right and exercise." We will take a closer look at the current thinking in terms of heart disease prevention and treatments. We will wrap up with a monograph on myths versus medicine and common pitfalls to avoid when trying to lead a healthy, happy lifestyle.

What This Book Is and Is Not

First and foremost, this book is not a substitute for anyone in need of individualized health care. It is not a substitute for consulting with your own physician on your own health needs. It is also not considered direct, personal medical advice. You should at all times seek advice from your own health-care practitioner.

This book is also not meant to be a comprehensive review of cardiovascular disease or its causes and effects. In fact, the term "heart attack" in some instances may not represent an exact definition of a heart attack. The term is often used as a metaphor for the emotional impact that any person might have in a stressful situation. So I beg your pardon and ask that you read with your eyes open and your thinking cap on. This book should in no way impair your need to investigate and explore heart disease on your own.

Finally, it is my intent to open, stimulate, and perhaps ease your mind as you think about this dreaded condition and begin to act deliberately to prevent it from afflicting you and your loved ones.

If you believe everything you read and hear, then I suggest you stop reading and stuff your ears with cotton.
-Coop-modified Japanese proverb

PART I
TRUTH

CHAPTER 1
THE FAMILY HISTORY

Genetics

Medicine has long since established that heart disease risk factors such as high blood pressure, high cholesterol, obesity, diabetes, cigarette smoking, and a lack of exercise put an individual directly at risk of developing heart disease. But what about genetics? What role does a person's genetic material play in the development of this deadly disease and its related conditions?

As it turns out, a family history has been shown to significantly increase the risk of developing heart disease. This is particularly true for men with a first-degree relative (parent or sibling) who develop heart disease before age fifty-five. In women, this statistic is slightly less negative (by degree), since their risk of developing heart disease is increased only if they have had a first-degree relative who developed heart disease prior to age sixty-five. Risk of heart disease for men and women is not only limited to those with siblings who have had a heart attack or coronary artery disease, but also those with relatives who have experienced a stroke or other major cardiovascular disease such as peripheral arterial disease. The subject of risk, as with many aspects of medicine, is much more involved than what I've presented here and will be fully explored in greater detail in Part II.

It is key for the reader to understand the influence of family history and genetics on heart disease development. This is precisely why I begin this book with my own family history, which is ironically chock-full of heart disease and other maladies.

It is also important to understand that while heart disease is particularly associated with a family history, so too are other diseases and conditions that include those listed as risk factors for heart disease. For example, high cholesterol levels in the blood (a risk for heart disease) are in some cases genetically inherited. Other diseases, notably the most common cancers of the breast, lung, and colon, are also related to inherited genetic material. Discussion of these in detail is beyond the scope of this book, but does bear mentioning and is important for the conveyance of my motivation for writing this book. I am dedicated to reducing the risk factors for heart disease that can be controlled. I believe that this can be done through education and increasing self-awareness, which, when applied directly to behavior, has the potential to save lives.

The Rock

The Missouri delta is where my journey began. Of course, the term "delta" is usually reserved for that portion of northwest Mississippi considered to be one of the lowest points in the continental United States. However, many people raised along the banks of the mighty Mississippi River have adopted "delta" to describe their home. This is particularly true for those born in the southern parts of Illinois, Missouri, Kentucky, and Tennessee, near the confluence of the Mississippi, Missouri, and Ohio Rivers.

Specifically, I was born in a small, rural agricultural town called Hayti (pronounced HEY-tie) in the southeastern boot-heel portion of Missouri. Although the spelling is similar to that of the country Haiti, there is no direct connection, except that the founders of Hayti, Missouri, modified the name "Haiti" to "Hayti."

I am the seventh of eight children born to the late Arthur Louise Cooper and Alex A. Cooper Sr. Large families are common among the Coopers. My father is one of eleven boys and one girl. Among his siblings, several have families of five or more children.

As one might expect, family gatherings are more like conventions. In fact, I am still meeting cousins, young and old, for the first time. Facilitated by the age of social media, I will on occasion get a

Facebook message with the familiar "hey cuz," to which I generally respond in kind, "hey cuz."

God, family, and education were the values espoused among the family. As educators, my parents naturally indoctrinated their children into their own core values. Education was the number-one priority in my family. Although I am a product of the local public school system, I credit much of my early education and academic success to those lessons learned at home. As children, we were expected to supplement our assigned reading in school with the classics such as *The Iliad* and *The Odyssey*. By middle school, I had read most of the Shakespearean classics.

I look back at these early, formative years of my life and feel overwhelmed with humility. I realize that I was very fortunate, that my parents worked very hard to provide me with every possible opportunity. Most importantly, they gave the kind of support that only deep love can. In our home, there were neither the necessities of life nor promises left unfulfilled. Christmas was the most anticipated and celebrated holiday. We always seemed to get more than we asked for and certainly more than we deserved. I am still not exactly sure how my parents managed to provide for all eight of us. My father tells me he never made more than fifty-two thousand dollars in a single year. I was embarrassed to tell him I have made that much in a month.

The strength in my family was the belief in dedication to family. Family was always at the core of most recreational and work-related activities. On Sunday afternoons we would all gather at my grandparents' farm in Missouri. Along with my siblings and extended family, I spent entire summers there working the land. The farm and the memories that have been built there continue to lure the current and succeeding generations. Each year for the past sixty-plus years, we have come together on the farm for a family reunion. It is held at the same time, on the same day—the second Saturday in August at noon. The roots of my family tree are strong and deep. I have been blessed with such a foundation.

What If? My Family, My Faith, My Medicine

As a physician now solidly in the prime of my career, I often contemplate the evolution of my life and the impact of my family upon it. And as this story unfolds, you too will see why I often ask myself the question, "What if?" What if things were different, and we could delay or interrupt the natural history of disease and the impact of one's family history upon it? This simple question leads me to contemplate my faith, my family, my education, and my commitment and passion for people and medicine.

The stories below represent a brief history of my own family history with respect to heart disease, illness, and the impact that these events have had on my personal and professional development. This history needs some introduction and a warning of sorts. Many aspects of these stories are very real and very sad. They are written to impart to you the different forms that heart disease takes, and the love for the people named in these stories that has driven my resolve to make a difference in the lives of others. As you will note in the following stories of my individual family members' health struggles, there are times in all of our lives when prayer is the only valuable final action.

Arthur Louise

As I am sure you are aware, large families are no strangers to death; this is simply a matter of statistics. In 1982, my mother died at the age of forty-six of pancreatic cancer. I was in the eighth grade and fourteen years old at the time. Thinking back to that time, I remember Mom frequently complaining of back pain. One day, I went in the bathroom after she had gone, and there was a pool of blood in the toilet. At that young age, I was curious and only thought that this was one of those "female things" that were beyond my scope at that point. I remember thinking perhaps she had just forgotten to flush. But now I know differently. The blood and chronic back pain were some of the classic signs and symptoms of the notoriously insidious pancreatic cancer. Eventually, she began to vomit incessantly due to bowel obstruction, and a trip to the doctor became unavoidable. When I later learned in medical school that what I was witnessing then were likely the beginnings of pancreatic cancer, I wondered, **"What if?"**

Vicki Renee

In 1997, my next-to-oldest sister, Vicki, called me from the University of Missouri Hospital in Columbia to inform me that she had a heart attack. For years, at this point, I was well into my training as a heart surgeon and offered any advice I could. Having essentially recovered from this initial insult to her heart, Vicki later moved to Atlanta to live with my family and me. She was suffering from the aftereffects of a weakened heart caused by her heart attack. The 1997 heart attack had caused her mitral valve to leak severely, which led to congestive heart failure (CHF—this condition will be explored in detail in later chapters). She needed surgery to correct this faulty valve. On September 7, 2001, she had this surgery at Emory Crawford Long Hospital, where I worked as staff surgeon.

The surgery was largely uneventful, and I left town the next day for a course in Salt Lake City, Utah. Everyone remembers that fateful day—September 11, 2001—but the next day is a date that will forever be ingrained in my memory. While stranded in Salt Lake City, I got the call from my colleagues that Vicki was in cardiac arrest, and they could not get her back. Vicki died that day from complications of the surgery.

For years prior to this, Vicki was given a diagnosis of asthma which was likely incorrect. The shortness of breath she was experiencing was likely due to heart disease. **"What if?"**

Leslie Nicole

Let's rewind to February of 1999, when I received a call that my youngest sister, Nicole, a beautiful young lady, was hospitalized in my hometown hospital in Hayti. At twenty-seven years old, she was given a new diagnosis of diabetes. Unfortunately, she had developed diabetic ketoacidosis, causing severe lung failure. Death was soon to follow.

As I think back on Nicole's short life, I remember her constantly drinking water and once even telling me that she always felt thirsty. This is called polydipsia, or excessive thirst, one of the classic signs of diabetes. **"What if?"**

Alvin Ardell

I was sitting at dinner with my father, wife, and a few friends on a Friday night in 2007 at the "Le Cabaret, Le Cabaret, Le Cabaret" formal event sponsored by the 100 Black Men of Atlanta. My cell phone began blowing up. I was getting call after call from family that I only rarely hear from or see except when someone dies. I began calling them back one by one until I finally got one of them, only to hear that my forty-five-year-old brother Alvin had just died of a massive heart attack.

Alvin was my closest sibling and served as best man in my wedding. He moved to Kansas City while I was there in medical school. I often spent weekends hanging out with him and his friends. He was a heavy smoker, and I remember he frequently complained of heartburn. He would literally chew on handfuls of Pepcid AC. Some years after I graduated and moved to Atlanta, Alvin moved to a small town in Arkansas. I got a call from him that he was hospitalized and was to undergo surgery to bypass a blocked artery (PVD—peripheral vascular disease) in his leg. This was some years prior to his death.

The combination of cigarette smoking, family history (recall my sister, Vicki Renee), heartburn, and PVD are all indications of coronary artery disease (CAD). The presence of CAD puts one at increased risk for heart attack. **"What if?"** I wondered.

These stories have been written to illustrate the power of knowledge to right, or at least mitigate, some of the suffering that these lovely people experienced. Let there be no mistake: our struggle is not with death. Our struggle is with life and how we live it. Our struggle is our faith, not just our faith in God, but our faith in our friends, family, and loved ones to help us in times of need. As Dr. Howard Thurman [6] reminded me in his book *The Creative Encounter* (1972), "There is nothing more searching in its exhilaration than the experience of meeting the need of another person at the point that the need is most acutely felt" (p. 107).

What I am most sincerely attempting to convey to you is the power of knowledge to potentially alter the course of events. There will be more about this concept later. Let us continue with the family history.

My father is the fourth son of Roy and Louise Cooper. There were twelve siblings in the family: eleven boys and one girl. Two of the Cooper men living to adulthood have passed on: my dad's oldest sibling Roy died in 2010 of congestive heart failure, which developed as a result of severe aortic stenosis (AS, which is discussed in Chapter 7), and the seventh son, Melvin (Uncle Fess), died in 2006 at sixty-nine years old of—you guessed it—a heart attack.

As you might imagine, all of the siblings have at least one or more of the common risk factors for heart disease, including high blood pressure, high cholesterol, and diabetes. One has even had a minor stroke (cerebrovascular disease). Interestingly, four have a condition called aortic stenosis—a narrowing of the aortic valve. Uncle Roy died of congestive heart failure (CHF) as a result of severe, untreated aortic stenosis, and three of the remaining siblings have a diagnosis of aortic stenosis.

Things don't get much better on my mom's side of the family. As I discussed earlier, she died a premature death (age forty-six) to metastatic pancreatic cancer. Her one and only sister died of lung cancer in her early sixties. Both my grandfather, Arthur Watson, and her dad died of a premature heart attack in his early sixties, and her mom lived into her late seventies, where she succumbed to a ruptured abdominal aortic aneurysm.

Much to Be Learned

Family history is one of the most powerful and helpful predictors of disease for any individual. Unfortunately, most of us, occupied by our day-to-day activities, fail to pause and contemplate how we came to be and how that can affect us in so many ways, physically and emotionally. It is my hope that by sharing my family story, you will not fall victim to "What if?" Hopefully, you will be inspired to engage on an active level in determining the status of your own health.

My family story is riddled with missed opportunities, passive dependency, and, in some cases, neglect. None of these should be chastised or ridiculed but on the contrary, put into perspective. If we had a little bit more of anything, I would only ask for a bit more communication among us all. Communication is so important because it opens the door to intervention.

Tell your story. By simply talking about what you are experiencing, you will form a more meaningful bond with your health-care provider and your family. Communication has three components: a message, a deliverer, and a receiver—not just a hearing receiver, but a true listener. I'm not suggesting that you reveal your most intimate health concerns to everyone you meet. However, you must but be willing to communicate with your doctor in order to get the most out of any healthy encounter. Tell your doctor your story, not just a few random symptoms: aches and pains, knocks, and pings. How do those symptoms and complaints fit into your daily life, how do they manifest themselves, and to what extent do they limit your quality of life? These are all important for you and your doctor to know.

Lean on your family a bit. There is someone out there who cares about you more than you do. Usually, that is a spouse or significant other. When faced with disease, the fear and anxiety associated with the unknown can be overwhelming for some. It is for this reason that it is so crucial to stay in communication with that special person who can be the facilitator who connects the dots. Likewise, you need to be willing to listen and empathize with those you love. Getting the best health outcome is a two-way street, and sometimes we are called upon to give, and not just receive, the caring hand.

Unplug and plug in to what's happening to you and your loved ones. I am often amazed at how powerful the need to be connected is. In the office, I usually give my patients plenty of time, but not infrequently, that time is interrupted by the ping, vibration, or ringing of an electronic device. Unplug when you sit down with your physician and demand that they unplug as well.

Second opinions help doctors too. From time to time I get the patient who is not convinced of my diagnosis and treatment plan. And often, they will apologize for wanting to seek the advice of another. News flash: it is often helpful to your physician to get a different perspective (and perhaps expertise) from someone other than themselves. So never be afraid to get a second opinion. In fact, I would be skeptical of any physician who did not encourage you to seek other advice when you would feel more comfortable doing so. Remember that your doctor may be thinking something, but won't say it to you for a number of different reasons. Alternatively, you both may be thinking the same thing, but neither has the courage to say so. When facing serious health concerns, don't play twenty questions. Say what's on your mind. The doctor's office has no stereotypes and should be a judgment-free zone. Doctors don't lie—we just sometimes struggle to tell the truth.

Here's another reason for communicating with your doctor every detail about what you do with regards to your health: that herbal supplement you're taking just might kill you. Certainly, I have a sincere respect for alternative forms of therapy. Sometimes I question the claims of such therapies, but when I see studies that refute the benefits of alternative therapies, I am just as likely to be skeptical. This is because most of these studies are designed to determine cause and effect, survival or death, or facilitation or prevention of disease. The methods chosen in these studies may not be designed appropriately. This does not invalidate these forms of treatment. We do not know what we do not know. On the other hand, traditional medicine has its place, and thus, I recommend that you not forgo the opportunity to cure for the unknown.

I've spent some time here emphasizing the importance of how your own family history may affect your health trajectory. I've also focused on the importance of acquiring knowledge related to conditions you may have and why you ought to communicate your thoughts, feelings, and experiences with your loved ones and your physician. Life is a long, collaborative event. At least, it should be. I often wonder if there had been more communication, a more active exchange of information within my own family and with family physicians, if outcomes would have been different. But today, the present, is what truly matters. I implore you to take these lessons to heart as we continue to explore these issues.

CHAPTER 2
THE HEART
OF A WOMAN

Overview

Although we know heart disease is the number-one killer of women and men, until recently heart disease was felt to be a "man's disease." But in fact, just as many women die of heart disease and heart attacks as men. If we include all forms of heart disease (including heart attacks), more women than men succumb each year [2]. Given the role that heart attacks and heart disease play in women's lives, a renewed focus on these issues is of utmost importance.

Heart disease and heart attacks in women have some unique characteristics that make education extremely important. Women must gain an understanding of the scope of these issues and identify related signs and symptoms of heart attack and disease in a timely manner, before damage becomes irreversible or worse. First, women often have heart attacks at an older age than men [2]. The reason for this phenomenon is thought to be the protective effect of estrogen on the heart in premenopausal women [2]. While the benefits of estrogen on premenopausal women may exist, women should be aware that this is not true for supplemental estrogen, which is oftentimes used in postmenopausal women. Supplemental estrogen in this population is not without risk; these women are at an increased risk of developing breast and ovarian cancer.

The importance of educating women cannot be overstressed. A 2006 Lifetime poll revealed the following discrepant information regarding women and heart disease [7]. Although more than half of women are now aware that heart disease is the number one disease threat, many still do not acknowledge their personal risk and do not routinely discuss the issue of risk with their health-care providers [8]. As one can see, knowledge and action are two very different things. While a person may know a certain thing, the motivation and inspiration to act may or may not follow. This is why education must be turned into action.

Another challenge women face is that the symptoms of heart disease can be quite different than those experienced by men. Women are also more likely to minimize those symptoms, and tend to be more concerned with the health of their loved ones than themselves. This stoic attribute in some women translates to reduced care. They are simply not getting the attention they deserve. Also, compared to men, women are more likely to have subtle, atypical symptoms such as heart palpitations, insomnia, shortness of breath, anxiety, fatigue, and generalized weakness [9]. These symptoms often go unnoticed because statistically, women are much less likely to report these symptoms to their doctors [9].

Lastly, and perhaps most impactful of all, diagnosis is often delayed in women. Health-care providers are less likely to suspect and thus detect heart disease in women, partly due to the female patient's stoic tendencies, generally speaking, and partly because of the atypical presentation of the symptoms. Another interesting fact that further muddies the water is that when properly diagnosed and treated, the treatments themselves may be more harmful for women. In one study, women undergoing coronary artery bypass surgery were found to have a risk of death two to three times higher than men [10]. This leads to what I call the Woman's Heart Triple Threat:

1. Lack of awareness/action
2. Atypical symptoms
3. Higher risk of complications with treatment

The Triple Threat to which women are subject is the number one reason for my writing this chapter. Of the three variables that comprise the Triple Threat, it is the first and second variables that education and action can affect. By working with women as physicians, as family members, and as friends, we are in a unique position to make real differences in the outcomes of women. Simply having a casual conversation with a family member may plant a seed of thought that later develops into real action when that individual realizes that the back pain she's experiencing may not, in fact, be back pain. My point is that every opportunity to educate has potential to achieve great results, even though these results may not be immediately apparent.

In my travels through this life, I have found that experience is the best teacher. Nothing beats having all of one's senses involved to make knowledge stick. With this in mind, I've compiled a number of stories from my practice to illustrate the signs and symptoms of how heart disease and heart attack present in women. This chapter explores these issues and the impact of heart disease and its related conditions on the lives of several women.

The Cover Girl

Serendipity or synchronicity brought Donna and me together. I affectionately refer to her as the "Cover Girl." This has been my nickname for her from the first time I saw her. She is a beautiful, blonde-haired, blue-eyed woman, married with children and living the American dream. She was not supposed to be lying on a gurney in my hospital on the night of November 3, 2007.

As a matter of fact, I was not supposed to be there either. At that time, I was actually on active duty and deployed to Fort Gordon in Augusta, Georgia, in support of Operation Enduring Freedom. I had been called up to backfill a position left open by a surgeon at Fort Gordon who had been deployed to Iraq. On that weekend, due to an unexpected issue, one of my Emory colleagues needed to make a switch in the call schedule and everyone else was unavailable. I was asked to come home for the weekend and cover call. Augusta is only a couple of hours away and so I agreed to do so.

I drove home the Friday night before that weekend to spend some time with the family. It was a quiet Friday evening. I got up the next morning and went in to make rounds without much clamor. After rounds, I headed home and spent the rest of the day hanging out with the family and a few friends. An uneventful day of call.

Later on that evening, I got a familiar phone call. The Kennestone Hospital Cardiac Catheterization Lab was on the line; Dr. Incorvati needed my assistance emergently. He was physically performing the heart catheterization procedure and could not come to the phone, so the nurse relayed the following information: a young, thirty-seven-year-old female was having a heart attack. A stent, which is a tube that props open an artery, was not feasible. She needed emergent open-heart surgery. I didn't need any more details than that to activate my team. I called the Heart Line and got the ball rolling. The Heart Line is a one-phone-call emergency system that activates the team on call with me to immediately come in and help.

I got in my car and headed to the hospital. Without traffic the drive was usually less than thirty minutes. As this is a frequent occurrence when on call, I had no particular thoughts about it. This was business as usual, unfortunately, as it is routine to get called in to perform emergency bypass surgery. The only unusual thing this time was the age of the patient, thirty-seven—not a typical emergent bypass patient.

When I arrived at the hospital, I was expecting to find a thirty-seven-year-old overweight diabetic with high blood pressure, maybe a family history of heart disease, and perhaps a smoker. But none the likeness thereof; Donna was as I described above. This was my first encounter with Donna. She was on the gurney headed into the cardiovascular operating room (CVOR) at Kennestone. Charita and my team were just about to move her onto the operating room table. She was surprisingly calm, not at all consistent with her poor vital signs—low blood pressure, pale, cold, and clammy. I have seen this before, just before the person dies. I rubbed her forehead and told her she was going to be okay. Although this action was meant to be comforting to me and the patient, God only knew what the outcome would be.

As we entered the CVOR, I found Dr. Chuck Lee, my cardiac anesthesiologist. We wasted no time in putting her to sleep and placing the breathing tube in her throat. During this procedure a large amount of pink, frothy fluid came up from the breathing tube. This is caused by a heart that is not pumping well, which leads to fluid accumulating in the lungs, a condition called pulmonary edema—a concerning sign.

As the team worked diligently to get her prepped and ready, Dr. Lee and I examined the heart with a trans-esophageal echo. This is a procedure where a fiber-optic scope is inserted into the esophagus, allowing close inspection of the heart and heart valves. The results were not good. Donna's heart was barely moving in the anterior area where her arteries were blocked. This was a dire situation and the reason for her pulmonary edema. Her heart was failing to pump, which caused blood to back up into the fine capillaries surrounding the lungs, and finally into her lungs. Time was of the essence.

I left the room to speak with the family. There they were, a "dying" husband and two beautiful girls in total distress. The desperation in their eyes was palpable. I could feel their despair. The thought of my family rushed through my mind. What would I do, how would I feel if I were him?

In a situation like this, the only strategy that I've found helpful is to underpromise and overperform. The worst thing a surgeon can do is give the family false hope. There are so many things that may go wrong with a heart attack. We do our best and pray for the best. This was especially tough since the two little girls reminded me so much of my two little girls of similar age at home. Mr. Fielding was literally begging me to deliver his wife, but I couldn't promise. I could only say that I would do my very best.

It was time to get to work. The team finished prepping and I started to open Donna's chest. Once in, it was obvious the heart was not moving. I did not have time to do my standard approach, which is to place the left internal mammary artery on the main artery on the front; a solution that allows for redistribution of blood to the area of the heart most in need. The heart was in such bad shape that I just needed to restore blood flow as quickly as possible. My PA took a piece of vein from the lower leg and we put that on to the main artery, called the left anterior descending (LAD) coronary artery, and one of its branches called the diagonal artery.

The LAD was extremely friable, meaning the tissue literally fell apart as I worked with it. This made the bypass of the blood vessel extremely difficult, since making attachments to vessels was that much harder than it typically already is. Upon closer inspection, I discovered that Donna had suffered a spontaneous dissection of the blood vessel (the LAD). She likely had an early atherosclerotic plaque in the area that lead to the tear, which then lead to a separation of the layers in the wall. We struggled to put this all back together.

Once we had this done, we had the same problem with the diagonal branch. Ultimately, we were able to get it finished. Unfortunately, Donna's heart was in very poor condition and not pumping well. I contemplated putting in a ventricular assist device (VAD), which would take over the work of pumping blood while her left ventricle recovered from this massive heart attack. I made the decision instead to give it time, waiting for a positive or negative trend to develop.

After a while, the miracle began to happen. Donna's heart began to recover right there in the operating room. It was enough recovery to allow us to wean her from the bypass machine without requiring the VAD. We closed her chest and took her to the intensive care unit. She was certainly in critical condition, but I was seeing the positive trend that I was looking for. In the end, Donna made a complete recovery and survived to tell her story.

At thirty-seven, the regular tennis player and mother of two healthy girls was as unlikely a heart attack victim as anyone could be. When the dust had settled, I delved a bit deeper into her story to uncover what had brought her to this point.

Upon closer inspection, there were signs for some time that things were not quite right. Several months before, in the spring of 2007, Donna noticed that she was more tired and fatigued than usual after a round of tennis. Subsequently, she developed jaw pain that lead to a root canal and crown replacement. She was also grieving the loss of her father, whose funeral was only days prior to her heart attack. In fact, during the memorial service, she became faint and EMS was called. Follow-up visits to the doctor revealed normal EKGs and blood work. Adding to the veil covering her underlying condition was Donna's physical appearance (young, healthy), certainly not enough to influence a decision to look further into the possibility of an underlying heart condition.

All along, Donna sought medical attention for subtle signs that are not typical of someone with a heart condition. Recognition of these subtle signs and rejection of the "healthy" stereotypes we often use to label based on appearances may have prevented Donna's heart attack. Her story reinforces the need for open communication not only from patient to physician and family, but among health-care providers. We, as physicians, must constantly remind ourselves that there is frequently more to every story. What appears to be the case may not be. Thankfully, she survived and now spends time volunteering and telling her story to others.

Me and Mrs. Jones

Several years ago, I was asked to see a sixty-year-old lady who had a stroke and was essentially paralyzed on her left side. The etiology of her stroke was an infection on her mitral valve; we call that particular disease state endocarditis. She had acquired the infection from a simple dental procedure some weeks earlier. The valve was destroyed and needed replacement. Before I walked into that room, I thought to myself, "I am not going to operate on this lady." Her stroke was too recent. The risk of another stroke was too high and would end it all.

I walked into the room and started talking to Mrs. Jones and her husband. Shortly after I began our conversation, I realized she could understand me but she could not respond. This is a phenomenon known as expressive aphasia, which is common after a stroke. I went through my talk about all the risks and benefits of surgery and why I think we should not do it.

As I finished, her husband looked up at me and said, "So when are we going to schedule the surgery?"

"Mr. Jones, I thought I was saying to you that I would not do surgery," I said.

"Let me tell you a story, Dr. Cooper," he said. "My wife and I have been together for some fifty years and we are in love." He went on to tell me about their love affair.

After Mr. Jones finished his story, I looked up and told him, "Mr. Jones, I will be honest with you. Before I came in this room, I had made up my mind that I would not operate on your wife. But as you spoke I began to wonder, what if?" I scheduled the surgery for the next day. Mrs. Jones did well during surgery, and the morning after I found her sitting in the chair at her bedside eating breakfast.

Some time later, I got a note from Mr. Jones thanking me for "believing and having faith in something other than my own ability and abstract knowledge from a book—that has never met Mrs. Jones and doesn't know God." He thanked me for giving him and his wife one more chance. Mrs. Jones died that same year of unrelated complications.

Mrs. Jones's story is an example of the importance of listening to your patient and the patient's family. Had I retained full control in the exchange between Mr. Jones and myself, the outcome may have been markedly different. As I've stated previously, we simply do not know what we do not know. Communication between doctor and patient, husband and wife, et al., is a wonderful and fundamentally crucial thing.

A Tormented Soul

She was a middle-aged, sixty years old or so, African American female. I had never met her before. I was consulted by another physician who wanted my input on her case and had to peruse her chart for a few minutes just to get information regarding the nature of her visit. As often occurs, the chart only told a minute portion of the story.

As I looked over the results of her tests, I was even more confused. Her heart catheterization showed relatively normal coronary arteries, and the echo showed that her heart function, although not normal, was not severely impaired. She had a stent placed into her left anterior descending artery during the last cath procedure.

As I was going about my usual Wednesday seeing patients in my office, I noticed her checking in. She was a woman of small stature and rather talkative as I walked by the vitals room. I introduced myself, shook her hand, and asked what brought her in to see me. Barely finishing my salutation, she let me know she was there to have another lead added to her pacemaker. The previous December, she had a biventricular pacer device placed transvenously, but the leads had poor capture. The referring physician sent her to me to have pacer leads placed directly on the heart. We have to do this infrequently when the transvenous leads do not function effectively. A word about this type of pacemaker: biventricular pacing is commonly done in patients with congestive heart failure to resynchronize the heartbeat and provide more efficient pumping in patients with heart failure. The symptoms of dyspnea (difficulty breathing) and shortness of breath can improve dramatically in some patients through biventricular pacing. However, as the interview continued, I could smell the aroma of cigarettes from her breath. She admitted continuing to smoke despite the fact that she was always short of breath and had been counseled against this in the past.

The stories began to flow. The more we talked, the more I realized this woman was not necessarily in need of my professional expertise on this day. She was really in need of prayer and comfort for her tormented soul. Her stress was palpable. She talked quite affectionately about a son in the navy who was coming to pick her up in late March. He did not want her to fly to New Orleans, so he planned to come to Georgia to pick her up. I could surmise that she was quite proud of him as she reflected on how comforting he was to her. Although she was his mother, he was like a father to her at this stage of her life.

It just so happened that she had nine children and twenty grandchildren. She was tormented by their lack of accomplishments in life, despite the fact that she had "raised them right" and "given them everything." They were constantly calling and demanding money. One daughter went so far as to threaten to kill her mother for not giving in to her demands for money. I learned there were other children with drug, money, and criminal problems. She could not understand why these things were happening to her. She was so distraught over the life choices of most of her children and her self-perceived failure that she had attempted suicide some years ago and was hospitalized as a result. This brought tears to her eyes and mine.

Periodically throughout our interview, she would refer to praying to God and being scared. She talked about praying to God to heal her heart, kidneys, and lungs. I was taken by this, but what I realized is that, at least in my interpretation, she was praying for the wrong things. It was obvious to me that what this lady needed more than healing of the physical was healing of the soul. After the suicide story, I stopped her and took both of her hands in mine and just asked her to be silent and be still. After several moments, I began to pray for her and asked God to heal her soul and remove the torment. We prayed together and finished our visit.

I walked out and finished my paperwork, and she went to the front desk. Some time later, after she had checked out, she asked for permission to come back to see me again. She walked up to me and, without speaking, she hugged me, said thank you, and left. I continued about my work, but also thanked God for using me as an instrument to deliver his words of comfort. Again, here was the power of communication.

An Angel in the Room

I received a call on a particular Thursday in late January of 2011. The call was no different than any of a number of calls I get throughout the day from referring physicians wanting to send patients for consultation or seeking advice on how to manage a particular problem with a patient. This was a request to see a middle-aged woman for possible aortic valve replacement surgery. The caveat in this case was the fact that she'd had two prior operations in the early 1990s for coronary artery bypass. A third operation could be a daunting challenge. The question was whether or not we should refer her out for an experimental procedure called percutaneous aortic valve replacement, or simply proceed with the traditional approach. Of course, I agreed to see her in consultation and began making arrangements for her to see me in my office the following week.

A peculiar thing happened the next day. I was summoned to the cath lab reading room to look at a cath film for another cardiologist. In the reading area there were several of our cardiologists sitting around preparing for the day's work ahead. One of those was the cardiologist I spoke to the day prior about the patient described in this story.

He began to tell me what happened after we ended our phone call the day prior. The patient began to cry and get very emotional when he mentioned my name, Dr. William Cooper, to her. He asked, of course, what was wrong. She went on to describe to him a near-death experience (NDE) she had while in the hospital in 2006. During that experience, she described to this cardiologist that she had met me previously, as an angel. She told him that when she had the cardiac arrest, I was one of several angels who appeared to her. He went on to tell the story, and of course I listened intently. I could sense the other doctors in the room thinking to themselves that perhaps the cardiologist, the patient, and I were all crazy. Not so at all, for I have learned to pay close attention and seek understanding even in the most peculiar situations.

The following week she came to see me in my office as scheduled. I walked in to meet her and her daughter and my first words were, "Ms. D, your angel has arrived." This surprised her and comforted her all at once, because she knew at that point that her doctor had spoken to me again and relayed her incredibly powerful story.

She then began to tell me her story. She described my frequently worn black shoes, socks, and slacks with a white coat and my entire persona surrounded by a "Shekinah" halo of glory, as she referred to it. I did not speak to her during her NDE, nor was I present during the event. However, she remembered quite vividly observing me talking to the cardiologist who was attending to her during her arrest. She recalled telling him, while in the state of cardiac arrest, that it was not time yet for her to have surgery.

Later that same day or perhaps the next, the cardiologist who attended to her during the cardiac arrest returned to her bedside to tell her about his real-life conversation with me. Before he could tell her he had spoken to me, she interrupted, "You spoke to Dr. Cooper and you have decided it is not time for me to have surgery." He wanted to know how she knew this; she was specific about him asking her three times to explain. She was hesitant to reveal how she knew but eventually relived the event for him. He was dumbfounded. Mrs. D was sure he thought she was crazy, or that somehow I had gone to see her. I, in fact, had never met this lady prior to her visit to my office.

I let her know that her story gave me comfort knowing that she felt I was an angel. Of course, I am not even one step close to being an angel, but as our elders sometimes say, God speaks to us in mysterious ways.

The following week we proceeded to surgery. As I expected, it was difficult. Each prior operation creates scar tissue in the healing process in place of normal, undisturbed tissues and structures, and she was no exception to this fact. We eventually got to the heart and were able to perform more bypasses, as well as replace the aortic valve.

Recovery from such an operation is no easier than the performance of the procedure. Both bleeding from the additional scar tissue and the overall function of the heart are of immediate concern post-operatively. We were fortunate in this case not to have problems with either of these two complications. However, she did develop kidney failure that required dialysis for several weeks after surgery.

Finally, things returned to normal for her, and she came into my office more energized than before, fully recovered and full of appreciation for a new lease on life. Having been a habitual smoker, this time, the cigarettes were gone. The effect of spiritual healing in conjunction with medical intervention cannot be dismissed as making a difference in our lives.

"Mom"

I affectionately refer to this patient as "Mom" because of her resemblance to my real mother. I have known Mom for over ten years. Our first encounter was chance and fate.

I met Mom's younger brother John first. In the early 2000s, John was admitted to Crawford Long Hospital for symptoms of congestive heart failure. Like so many young African American men, John was overweight with high blood pressure and high cholesterol. The underlying cause of his heart failure was a leaky aortic valve and an ascending aortic aneurysm, in addition to other factors. John needed surgery to correct the problem.

The day I went to see John, he was alone in his room. He was a burly, fair-skinned man, quiet and soft-spoken. I went over the problem that led to his condition and my treatment plan, which included open-heart surgery to replace the valve and the aneurysm. John understood and agreed to proceed with surgery.

As I was making rounds that evening, one of the nurses stopped me to inform me that John's sister wanted to speak to me about his surgery. She wanted to know, "Who is this Dr. Cooper and what are his credentials?" I was slightly taken aback, but told the nurse to call me when John's sister showed up so that I could come and meet her in person and go over the surgical plan with her.

Later that evening we had our meeting. I went to John's room but found only John. As I walked out, down the hall was this beautiful, salt-and-pepper-haired black woman of tall stature, well-dressed and professional-looking, walking toward me. I introduced myself and found that she was John's sister. Wow! She had such a striking resemblance and reminded me of my own mother. She was exquisitely professional, well-spoken, and classy.

We returned to John's room and, in his presence, I went over his condition and our surgical plan in great detail. She had lots of questions, not the least of which was about my surgical credentials. At the time I was fairly fresh out of training, but this was an operation that I had already performed on numerous occasions. I learned that she worked as an administrator in Fulton County government. She was an important person with important connections and I knew it. However, all of my patients are just as important, and I was going to give John the same attention and care that I gave all of my patients. They deserve it and we deliver it every day.

I operated on John the next day. He required an aortic valve replacement and repair of an ascending aortic aneurysm. The surgery went well. John recovered and went home a few days later. That did not end my relationship with "Mom," as I discovered during John's ordeal that she and I attended the same church in southwest Atlanta—Cascade United Methodist Church. Over the ensuing years, we would often talk after church service. John did well from his heart surgery, but he developed esophageal cancer and died a few years later. Mom took it all in stride, as she did during his open-heart surgery. She was grateful for my care of John.

Mom was in good physical condition. As our relationship developed, she opened up about her health challenges, which among other concerns, included high blood pressure. After church one Sunday morning in the fall of 2010, Mom tracked me down to ask a question. She recently had her annual physical and had a concern about the report from her doctor. She was not clear on the details, so I told her to get an appointment in my office for a second opinion.

After reviewing her records and the echocardiogram, it was obvious Mom had a serious problem. Despite exercising and feeling well, the echocardiogram revealed a leaky aortic valve and an ascending aortic aneurysm—the same condition that I treated for her brother John.

The extent of an aneurysm was unclear on the echocardiogram, as is usual, so I ordered a CT angiogram to get a better look. Indeed, the aneurysm was quite large. However, it was not of a size that warranted immediate surgery, so I scheduled her for a follow-up surveillance exam and CT scan. She returned in six months with a scan that showed the aneurysm had grown substantially, and the leakage from the aortic valve had gotten worse. It was time to consider surgery.

For most patients in good health, the decision to proceed with open-heart surgery can be difficult. This was the case with Mom. She exercised every day and felt well, but the tests were undeniable. She had to make a decision.

She agreed to proceed. In early June of 2011, we went to surgery. I was expecting to find the usual, an aneurysm and leaky valve, but there was more. Mom had a healed, chronic aortic dissection. An aortic dissection is caused by high blood pressure and is particularly common in the setting of an aortic aneurysm. It is usually an undeniable condition to diagnose because when it occurs, it causes a tearing chest discomfort that forces the victim to seek immediate medical attention. If not treated immediately, the vast majority of patients will die within a few hours or days. Mom was lucky she survived this long with a life-threatening condition. It is unclear when it actually occurred, as it was not obvious on the scans and x-rays.

I had seen this before and we were prepared to handle the situation. We completed the operation by performing a valve-sparing aortic root replacement. In simple terms, the leaky valve that was caused by the aortic dissection was actually a normal valve and did not need to be replaced. We left it in place and got rid of the aneurysm and dissection.

Mom recovered from surgery and did well. She continues to exercise every day and maintains a healthy weight. Her high blood pressure was initially very difficult to control, however, with exercise, weight loss, and medication adjustments, it is now consistently normal. We have maintained our relationship and follow-up scans of her aorta look totally normal. Mom's personality was what saved her. Her forwardness and willingness to assert herself to someone she trusted brought her condition to light in time for an intervention.

***

As I stated in Chapter 1, there is one common beginning place from which the door is opened to healing in every individual. This is communication. We are given a brain to interpret and evaluate our way through life. We are also given a mouth and the emotional push to use it. The stopping point, the reasons for not communicating our needs are many, some of which cannot be overcome except for internally. But they must be overcome. In the success stories of health care, survivors often share the ability to ask for and get what they most require. And in cases where a person cannot speak for themselves, if family knows this person's needs, the patient has a fighting chance. Communication is the key.

CHAPTER 3
ZAMINA AND NINETY
DAYS IN THE CSH

I have had the honor and privilege of serving in the Army Reserve since 1985. When I signed up on January 19, 1985, I never thought I would be deployed and serve in a real combat situation. No one ever does. But the world has changed and is changing right before our eyes. And I certainly never thought I would be dealing with heart attacks or heart-related issues while serving. Perhaps it is the nature of what I do that attracts the heart attack to me.

Indeed, while serving in Iraq in 2003 and Afghanistan in 2010, I was confronted with the dreadful heart attack. After my Iraq experience, I decided to record in detail the experience of my next overseas deployment, which came in the early spring and summer of 2010.

One story is that of a seemingly healthy soldier who had a heart attack while serving as a doctor in the same combat support hospital (CSH) as I. Zamina's story although not a classic "heart attack" evoked a lot of emotion not just from me, but many of the physician soldiers caring for her during that time. Rather than retelling the story, I have included it here as firsthand accounting of the events related to her.

Day T-29, Wednesday, July 7, 2010

Today was an interesting but tiring day. I spent all day in the operating room (OR) with Paul Phillips. We did an ORIF (open reduction internal fixation, used by orthopedic surgeons to fix broken bones) of a left humerus fracture with repair of the radial nerve. This was stuff I had read about in my distant medical past but had never actually seen since residency, or, correction, since my tour in Iraq. Our second case was a rodding of the right femur and washout of several wounds. I kind of enjoyed the cases. Paul is a good surgeon and easygoing. Hmm, might think about orthopedics one day when CT (cardiothoracic) surgery is all dried up. Ha, yeah right.

Things got more interesting when our new DCCS (Deputy Commander of Clinical Services) Bob Haney got sick after exercising. We kept hearing about it as people were passing through the OR. It sounded like he was dehydrated as a lot of us get out here from time to time. PJ took over the job of DCCS for a while, and boy was he excited. He kept reminding everyone, "I'm the new DCCS." Some people have a need to be in a position of "authority." The DCCS job is more like psychosocial worker, dealing with patient logistics and answering the nagging questions. Knock yourself out, PJ.

However, it turned out that Bob was actually having a heart attack. He came back later and did more blood work, and indeed, he was having a heart attack. His electrocardiogram (EKG) had changed significantly from the first one he took earlier in the day. Peter Taillac was taking care of him and was a bit upset that he did not recognize it earlier. I reminded him that the vast majority of heart attacks present atypically, meaning without classic symptoms.

Bob was transported out by critical care air transport (CCAT) around one o'clock in the morning. He was stable but having a lot of arrhythmias. I certainly hope he does well; we should get some information soon.

Day T-28, Thursday, July 8, 2010
Then we got busy. Around 1:30 p.m., we got the call; an errant round (shot by us) hit a local bazaar. We had reports of as many as twenty-five casualties. Of course, everyone was running around trying to get prepared, but many were quite anxious. This was the

first time I have heard the phrase "Liberty Sally," meaning that we really don't know how many people we are getting and that all first responders and medical personnel, whether assigned or not, are to report to the Combat Support Hospital (CSH). "Sally" is a holdover from the days when the incoming casualties were called "mustangs," for Mustang Sally.

Reportedly, one of our 155 rounds went off course and took out a bunch of civilian noncombatants. So here we go. My patient was hit in the "box." This is the area between and below the nipples. I put my finger in the hole and I could feel his heart beating on the tip. Basically, an injury in this area requires surgery. I put a tube in his left chest and we intubated him and took him to surgery. I opened his left chest and got out a lot of blood. Indeed, the shrapnel had hit his heart and left lung. The heart was not through the muscle, but it took out a good chunk. The lung I repaired with a running stitch in the area. As I was about to finish this part, his heart essentially stopped, so I carried my incision all the way across his chest to gain full access and to search for an obvious cause. Unfortunately, the damage was done before he got to us. The wound on the heart was too near the major blood vessel on the front, the LAD, and this clotted, causing a heart attack. Back home, we may have been able to salvage the situation, but here, we could not afford to expend any more resources on this man. He died in the operating room a minute later.

I was proud of the team; they had come a long way and did a good job without too much chaos.

Day T-21, Thursday, July 15, 2010

Well, it was a slow day until about 9:30. We got a call, once again, from the local Khost hospital wanting to send us two patients. This is rather typical, as Friday is the "holy day" and no one wants to work on Fridays. Ah, I have seen this type of behavior before back home. There is a pattern in which some docs will call you on Friday afternoon with the "patient can't wait" transfer.

This time, it was reportedly a mortar round aimed at us that went off course and hit a family's home. We got two little girls, one four, and the one I took care of, seven. This happened around 11:30 in the morning and it took them all day to figure out they needed us. I took care of the seven-year-old little girl. She had already been operated on at the other hospital. Unfortunately, they missed the hole in her back that went into her left lung and, on the way, hit her spine, paralyzing her from the waist down. We also reexplored her abdomen and found that they had missed a hole in her bowel opposite the one they did repair. We also drained the blood from her left chest with a tube and took her to the ICU. She will survive but will be paraplegic.

Her little sister was hit in the pelvis and bladder. She also needed repeat surgery. Paul and McGraw did that surgery. She did well also. We later found out that the mother and another sister did not fare so well. They were both killed in the attack.

Day T-20, Friday, July 16, 2010

We finished the cases last night around 1 a.m. and did our usual rounds and clean up this morning. I did not work out this morning.

As I sit here writing in this journal, we are under missile attack. About thirty minutes ago, I heard a loud boom; since then, they are repeatedly announcing overhead to stay in the bunkers. Fortunately, our rooms are our bunkers; they are made of two-feet-thick concrete. Thank GOD! So far, we have not been called to the hospital.

Day T-17, Monday, July 19, 2010

The day began early. Bahktzamina, our seven-year-old with paraplegia, got into trouble early this morning. Her right lung completely collapsed due to a mucus plug. This is fairly common in a patient with a spinal cord injury. PJ and I struggled with her for several hours from about 1:00 until 3:00 this morning. We had to reintubate here (reinsert the breathing tube) and do bronchoscopy.

We eventually got her off the ventilator. We both recognized that this is going to be a long-term problem for her and will likely lead to her demise.

So that was the morning, and the evening was much more chaotic. Paul, Greg, PJ, and I were sitting on the roof when we got a call for an Afghan National Army soldier who had been hit with shrapnel to his hand and thigh area. We joked about how silly it seemed to send a helicopter to get him for what seemed like a non-life-threatening injury. And by the way, it costs six thousand dollars an hour to run a medevac helicopter, and they always travel in pairs. To sum it all up, a minimum of twelve thousand tax dollars an hour for what at the time did not seem like an emergency.

This one went from a silly situation to a really bad one in a hurry. A few minutes later they called back to tell us that they were bringing a total of four patients, including an additional three US soldiers in the same area who were involved in a roll-over vehicle accident but were all ambulatory at the scene. Okay, no problem, bring them in.

I would say about thirty minutes went by and another call came in. This time, one of the medics who was dispatched with the helicopter medevac had fallen while trying to extract one of our ambulatory (walking and talking) soldiers in a hoist and was tossed into a rocky cliff, sustaining a possible broken femur. More information flowed in and the soldier was identified as a female medic who was well known to all of the team. Indeed, the situation was now very serious. This was one of our best medics who went out on a routine medevac that was probably not necessary in the first place and came back on a backboard with a broken leg. It was badly broken in three places. I helped Paul wash out her knee and we put an ex fix (external fixation) on her femur fracture. This will basically end her flight medic career.

To add insult to injury, the medic on the ground was hit in the head by the hoist that the other medic was attached to. He was now on his way to see us with a head and neck injury. Luckily, his CT scan did not show any injury, but he did sustain a bad neck strain. Even more ridiculous was the fact that the four patients that we went after in the first place were now not coming because they were not injured enough to justify the trip.

I later learned that the medevac helicopter, while attempting to do the hoist, got into trouble (almost crashed as it was too close to the ground) and had to pull up. The female medic who was attached to the hoist was then flung into the medic on the ground, hitting him in the head and breaking her leg.

The sum total of all of this is absolute insanity. A medevac is dispatched unnecessarily and a risky extraction with a hoist was attempted, severely injuring one medic, nearly severely injuring another medic, and almost crashing a helicopter—for four patients with minor injuries, who, after the dust cleared, probably did not require the medevac in the first place. And so the drumbeat of war rolls on.

Day T-16, Tuesday, July 20, 2010

I got a call early again this morning around 4:30 a.m. I was struggling to get out of bed. Little Zamia's morning chest x-ray showed collapse of her lung again. This time it was the left lung.

Again, we intubated her and did bronchoscopy. We got the same thing, a lot of mucus plugs. This is a problem. She is not strong enough due to her paraplegia to cough, breathe deeply, or clear her secretions normally. Of course, we are all concerned about this. In this country with very limited resources, her lifespan has been severely reduced. If this had occurred at her village home, she would not have survived.

Day T-15, Wednesday, July 21, 2010

We made rounds and had a long discussion about what to do for and with Zamina. There are no good options. I readily admit to my selfishness in that I am glad I will likely not be here to decide her ultimate fate. I am redeploying in a couple of weeks and she will probably still be here.

I did another bronchoscopy on her today and discovered that the secretions are too abundant for us to extubate her. I will repeat it again this afternoon and continue repeating it until things look better; only then will we consider removing the tube again.

Zamina's bronchoscopy looked better this afternoon. I am hopeful that we will make progress over the next few days.

Day T-14, Thursday, July 22, 2010

I just finished the bronchoscopy on Zamina. Again, we got a lot of thick secretions. Her chest x-ray is also showing signs of an enlarging effusion on the left side. I will probably have to put a chest tube back in her at some point. This is getting more and more frustrating each day. I remain determined to do all I can for her.

Day T-13, Friday, July 23, 2010

We had a long discussion about what to do with little Zamina this morning. She had a large pleural effusion on the left side of her chest on this morning's x-ray. We all got together to discuss the options. In the States, this conversation would not have occurred because we have and will expend all the necessary resources to take good care of a paraplegic child. It happens every day in the US. However, here the challenges are significant. First of all, in the CSH hospital, we have a limited number of beds (eight) with the primary intent to take care of injured US soldiers. Along with the limited number of beds comes a limited number of personnel to care for those injured. We also operate on the assumption that all of our US casualties will be transferred to a higher echelon of care within a few hours of stabilization.

Here now we have a paraplegic female child with no mother and no female caregiver to look after her once she does leave the hospital. But before we get to discharge, how far are we willing to go with her lung issues? She has a very weak cough and is physically very weak in general because of her injury. Do we keep her on the ventilator for an extended period of time? If she is not able to mobilize her own secretions, do we do a tracheostomy and escalate the level of care? After a long discussion with everyone expressing their various opinions, the consensus was to continue to do all we can for her. Our commitment to this child is not based on the type of injury she had, but on our ability to care for whatever the injuries might be. So we remain committed to do all we can to get her better.

I took Zamina to the OR this morning to put the chest tube back in on the left side. We drained almost a liter of fluid from that side. I did another bronchoscopy and it actually looked good. In the early afternoon, we were able to extubate her again, and so far she is doing well. We are finally getting her and her caretaker to understand the importance of coughing and deep breathing. She was even able to suction herself.

We have yet to see the father, only uncles. The Afghan people live communally in their villages. The men dominate and the women in this culture are considered subordinate. They are not allowed in public without cover and are not allowed to speak to or be seen by a man other than the husband. It would be criminal in this society to address a man's wife directly.

Day T-8, Wednesday, July 28, 2010

Okay, back to Zamina: her lung is collapsed again. We had four good days and now this. The good news is that clinically she was doing well. We only detected this on the morning's chest x-ray. I took her to the OR to put in another chest tube and do bronchoscopy. Actually, the bronchoscopy was the best I have seen in her since admission. The chest x-ray afterward showed the lung reexpanded and the tubes in good position.

I have to ask myself why this continues to occur in her. I am suspicious that the bullet that is still in the lung or left chest is somehow responsible for this. If we see no improvement over the next couple of days, I may have to do a thoracotomy on her and explore the chest to see what's going on in there.

Day T-7, Thursday, July 29, 2010

As I suspected, the chest tube maneuver did not work. After a long debate with PJ and Pat about whether or not to get a CT scan on her, we ended up taking her to the operating room. The chest x-ray, which is what I wanted to see, showed again the collapse of the left lung. When something is not quite right, as most surgeons know, the best thing to do is explore.

The fragment from the bomb blast had penetrated her lung and rested inside the segmental bronchus to the superior segment of the left lower lobe. PJ and I debated about how to deal with this. Back at home, I would have done a formal segmentectomy (removal of a lung segment, or portion of the lung) of this part of her lung. In this setting, we opted for the more conservative approach. I opened the lung and cut right down on the fragment, pulled it out, and closed the hole in the bronchus. I also did a mechanical and chemical pleurodesis with doxycycline. The operation went well. We even let the commander scrub in and touch the little girl's heart. He has been struggling with his decision to bring her here. I think the exercise was therapeutic for him.

The rest of her day was benign. We got her off the ventilator quickly after surgery, and the evening after that was peaceful.

Day T-6, Friday, July 30, 2010

Our little Zamina had a reasonable night. I got one call on her around midnight. She had developed an air leak from one of her chest tubes, but she was doing well on her own. The morning's chest x-ray indeed showed a small pneumothorax, but otherwise the lung was well inflated. She is also developing some skin breakdown on her sacrum. She is paraplegic and has to rely on nursing to turn her often and get her out of bed and off her butt to reduce the pressure.

Zamina is our only patient this morning. She is doing well. I got a chance to meet her father for the first time. He was very thankful for all we had done. He wanted to know if she would be able to walk again. I had to tell him that that is very unlikely. He was still appreciative and wanted us to keep her here as long as it takes to get her well. Unfortunately, that does not mean she will ever regain use of her legs.

Friday, August 6, 2010

Little Zamina will go home today. Everyone is excited about the fact that she moved her left leg yesterday. Her chest x-ray is the best I have seen in quite some time. We will DC (discontinue) the tube and let her go home with her family. They just arrived here.

Friday, August 20, 2010

I am officially done with my outprocessing now and just returned home for the last time, for now, from Fort Benning.

I got another email report on Zamina. She has had several return visits to the CSH and continues to do well. We don't always know what our true purpose is in certain situations, but we should always maintain our faith and trust that GOD will always bring us home.

CHAPTER 4
ALL THE KING'S MEN

It would be a grave injustice to write a book about heart attacks and not include a section dealing with men. I won't repeat all of the things I have already said about heart attacks specifically for men, for as I am sure you are aware, the majority of what we know about the disease has been studied in middle-aged Caucasian men. Unfortunately, this puts other groups such as women and minorities at a disadvantage when it comes to extrapolating data from a large majority population to these subgroups. Nonetheless, the experiences of men with heart attacks are no less important than anyone else. In this chapter I will share a few lessons learned from some of those men.

The Captain

Before I met the Captain, I had been contemplating writing a book about heart disease and the many lessons it has taught me as a heart doctor and my patients who have succumbed to it. That contemplation turned to a yearning desire shortly after I met the Captain. He was a large white man, at least six feet four inches tall, with silver-gray hair and glasses. He had a rather deep, distinguished voice and he spoke with clarity and intelligence. And as you might imagine, his conversations were captivating and all the while informative as he spoke of his ordeals with heart disease.

I call him "the Captain" because he flew jumbo jets internationally for years with Delta Airlines. When I first met him, he was retired, partly due to his heart disease. His difficulties had begun at another hospital in town several years prior to our meeting. He had a heart attack and, as a result, underwent multiple stents to his coronary arteries to treat the blockages. He was told the stents would be good for a long time and he would be "okay." Not so fast.

Not long after his first heart attack and the stents, he was admitted to my hospital with another heart attack. The stents were blocked and could not be opened after multiple attempts by one or our interventional cardiologists. I was called to consider bypass surgery for him. This was not a pretty picture, for lack of a better way to put it, as his arteries were extensively calcified, small, and the stents were literally lining the vessels from start to near the end. This was not good, for the bypass surgery would require a place to sew the blood vessels together. Stents along the course of the vessel cannot be removed or sewn onto. This creates a difficult problem for the heart surgeon, who has to try to work around the blockages and the stents. I was not optimistic about my ability to help the Captain. I was willing to give it a try, but I would make no promises about the outcome because I simply did not know how bad it would be.

Of course, the Captain took the news quite ostensibly with no fear of the unknown but much animus toward the prior cardiologist for not being forthright with the extensiveness of his coronary artery disease and calcification of his blood vessels. The Captain felt betrayed.

I was there to help and I was determined to do all I could to get him back to health. Although I knew my chances were not good, it's the only chance he had.

After a long discussion with the Captain that evening, we prepared him for surgery the next day to bypass his blocked arteries. Yes, it was as bad as it looked on his heart catheterization the day prior. The coronary arteries were small and heavily calcified throughout their entire course. On top of the calcium and hardened arteries, stents lined the vessels making it difficult to find an area to bypass. We struggled through it and did the best we could. I planned to do four bypasses but could only do two. Despite this, the Captain tolerated the procedure well and made it out of the operating room just fine.

The Captain continued to recover over the ensuing days. His mood and outlook improved every day. I think he gradually began to accept his condition and take it head on. I enjoyed spending time with and talking to him. He had many stories of his flying days and other days as well. But now it was time to turn the page and focus on the things he could do to improve his health and not dwell on those things which could not be changed. The fact of the matter is despite his frustration with having been given a clean bill of health by his prior doctors, his heart disease was largely a result of his lifestyle. He had lived well.

As has been the case on many occasions throughout my career, toward the end of his stay in the hospital, I felt like I had a new friend and not necessarily a patient. I never take this for granted and I never forget how vulnerable my patients are as they battle with heart disease. On the other hand, sickness creates a most captive audience and never will the influence of a doctor be more impactful than at the patient's point of greatest need.

On his last day in the hospital as I was leaving the room, the Captain called me back in for one more "thank you." As he shook my hand one more time, he said, "Doc, I think you should write a book. You have a story to tell and there are people who need to hear it." By this time, after many visits from me and many conversations, he had become familiar with just about everything about me, including my family history. It was no surprise that he would say this. I paused there for a moment and thought to myself, *You know what, Captain? You are right. I should write a book.* So here's to you, Captain. Thanks for the inspiration and the bottle of Jordan.

The Patriot

Our contemporary political climate is nothing short of miserable divisiveness. I often chuckle at the so-called "politically incorrect" media using terms such as "patriot" and "great American," as if

41

they have somehow distinguished themselves from the rest of us by their vernacular. I chuckle, because during my time in the military I have met some of the finest Americans ever known to this great country of ours.

One of those great Americans walked into my office in the spring of 2008. I call him "the Patriot." Keep reading and you will find out why.

As I have for years, I hold my office hours on Wednesday mornings. The day the Patriot came in was just another ordinary day. There was just one peculiar thing as I perused my schedule for the day; I noticed there was one patient on the list that was an eighteen-year-old. It was peculiar because I don't usually treat eighteen-year-olds and I don't do pediatric heart surgery. So why was this person on my schedule? I would soon find out.

As the Patriot came in to the office exam room, I noticed he and his mother walking through the clinical area. He did not appear to have any heart condition. His mother was not far behind and I heard her ask the nurse as they walked through, "Is that Dr. Cooper?"

The nurse replied, "Yes."

Still curious, I looked up and said, "Hello, I will be with you shortly."

I completed my paperwork on the prior patient and walked in to meet the Patriot and his mother, who almost immediately came undone and began to cry and thank God. I was now getting a bit anxious because I barely got out another "hello" before the wailing started. The Patriot sat quietly and shook my hand. Eventually he had to ask his mother to pipe down.

She went on and on about how God had sent them to me to heal her son. She saw an article about me in the local newspaper and she was convinced I would save her son. At this point, the son did not look like someone who needed saving, as he looked perfectly healthy to me.

Once we got Mom calmed down, he began to tell his story. He graduated from a local high school in Marietta, Georgia, and enlisted in the navy. He wanted to be a Navy Seal and that's all he wanted to do. He decided before he signed up that if he could not be a candidate for Seal School then he would be allowed to be discharged from the navy to do something else. I was really surprised at this, but there it was in black and white: a letter from the navy commandant stating as much, that if he was not qualified to become a Seal then he would be discharged, and indeed he was.

After the Patriot finished basic training in Great Lakes, Michigan, he went on to begin his qualification for the Seals. During his physical examination, which is quite extensive, the chest x-ray showed an abnormality. This x-ray was followed up with a CT scan of his chest, and he was found to have a pericardial mass that appeared to be a pericardial cyst. Pericardial cysts are benign incidental findings often seen on cat scans and x-rays of the chest. They don't usually require surgical treatment unless the diagnosis is unclear or they are large and compressing other vital structures. Neither of these were true for the Patriot.

Unfortunately, the navy was uncertain what impact this would have on the Patriot's Seal training and thus he was disqualified. He could not convince the navy surgeons to remove the cyst so it would not interfere with his training. They would not do it.

The Patriot was determined, so he made another smart move. He got the navy to agree to allow him to return to be re-examined and reconsidered for Seal training if he could find a civilian surgeon to remove the pericardial cyst. Once again, I was in disbelief until I saw the letter stating the facts. Indeed, he would be allowed to return if the issue of the cyst was resolved.

No problem, Patriot! You came to the right place. Dr. Cooper was not going to allow this to get in the way of a committed young man's dream of serving his country. The navy surgeons forgot the other indication for surgery in cases like this. The cyst was interfering with the young man's occupation. Yes, at times, health issues get in the way of us doing our jobs and fulfilling our dreams. If surgery can correct the problem, then surgery it is.

After hearing this story, I was ready and willing to do all I could to get the Patriot back on track. Imagine this. He had the foresight to ask for a release if he was disqualified and recon-sideration if he could get it fixed. This was such an inspiring story. I must admit, if I had not seen the trail of paperwork, this would have been difficult to believe.

I removed the Patriot's pericardial cyst the next week. The surgery was simple and straightforward. It took only twenty minutes to complete.

He returned to see me after a couple of weeks and, despite my instructions to the contrary, he was already doing 100 plus pushups and sit ups each day. He was eager to begin swimming and get a release to return to the navy. I did even more. I wrote a letter to the commandant recommending that the Patriot get an immediate reconsideration to return to the navy for Seal School. Three months later, the Patriot was back in the navy, on to BUD/S (a program for candidates for Seal Training), and then formal Seal Training. He became a Seal in 2010.

His mother gives me a call from time to time to let me know he is doing well. You can't just reach out and hit him on his cell. Every time I see our fighting men and women around the world, I think of him. I know he is out there, stealth, quiet, invisible, lurking after our enemies. Protecting our asses from the violence of terror. He stopped by the office on a couple of occasions over the years. The last time he dropped off a hat with "Seal Team 8" on it. This, my friends, is a true patriot.

PART II
TRAGEDY

CHAPTER 5
THE PERFECT PUMP

The Origins of a Killer

Before 1900, very few people died of heart disease. Take a moment to think about this statement. I can remember my grandmother reminiscing of homemade cream pies. Yes, a cream pie, which is a decadent and serious dessert with three very heavy-hitting ingredients: cream, sugar, and eggs. Her mother would also bake her own bread in the evenings. The family would gather around the still-warm oven and slather butter all over that bread. In the mornings, there would be milk that had been delivered to the front doorstep. This was no lightweight milk; not 1 percent, 2 percent, or heaven forbid . . . skim. No, this was real, whole milk with an obscene layer of cream on the top. My grandmother's fondest memory was that rare occasion when she would get to take the cream off the top for herself.

I will stop this line of storytelling before I make my readers cry. What has happened since that time? Why has heart disease become the number-one killer in the United States? With all that fat in the diet, why is this disease and its related conditions a leading cause of death in the United States?

One answer lies in one of humanity's greatest advances, the Industrial Revolution. In the short span of less than one century, the majority of the civilized world radically changed the way that it lived, worked, and played. Daily life in the pre-industrial world was hard. The majority of people made their living through some sort of manual labor. Walking was the major means of transportation. Laundry was scrubbed and wrung by hand. Stairs were climbed, carpets were beaten, and butter was churned. As technological advances slowly became a part of everyday life, the daily life of each individual was gradually transformed. It became generally easier as most manual labor was either replaced or assisted by machinery. Automobiles, washing machines, elevators, and vacuum cleaners became commonplace. Machines were built to homogenize milk, process cheese, churn butter, and make ice cream. These modern conveniences made physical activity unnecessary and, in many instances, unwanted.

Along with the change in lifestyle came a change in diet. Grains began to be produced by methods that increased their availability to the general public. Advances in food delivery also made food more easily accessible. Along with this increase in food choices came increases in quantity and, oftentimes, decreases in quality. Luxury foods, like fried foods, potato chips, hamburgers, and french fries, became common additions to everyday meals (in some cases replacing meals entirely).

It was this deadly combination of a sedentary lifestyle and a rich diet that led to an increase in clogged blood vessels, heart attacks, and strokes among the population. Heart disease became commonplace. In fact, the rate of heart disease increased so sharply between 1940 and 1967 that the World Health Organization called it the world's most serious epidemic. A killer was born.

Medical science immediately went to work studying the disease and searching for its causes and cures. A thirty-year study of this issue (started in 1948) began in Framingham, Massachusetts. The Framingham Study involved 5,127 people aged thirty to sixty-two who showed no signs of heart disease [12]. Every two years, these participants underwent a complete physical examination. The study lasted thirty years and provided priceless profile information for predicting heart disease. This study and others like it were the beginning of an acknowledgment within the medical culture that there was indeed something happening to the population. Something was shortening lives and weakening people in a manner which followed a previously unseen trend. That something was heart disease.

The Pump

In its pure, unmolested state, the human heart is an extremely efficient and remarkable thing. Before arteries are clogged (stenotic), before cardiac muscle is damaged (a side effect of a heart attack), the pump works like it just rolled off of the factory floor. But you may be wondering how this miraculous machine, about the size of a fist and weighing in at between nine and twelve ounces, works. I'm going to attempt to make this explanation as straightforward and meaningful as possible. This is because I believe it important for readers without a medical background to grasp the fundamentals, without which trying to understand the heart in greater detail becomes nearly impossible. So, allow me to give a tutorial that I think you'll find reasonably simple.

Think of the heart as two small single-chamber pumps, the atria, sitting on top of two larger single-chamber pumps, the ventricles. The heart is then divided into the left and right side. The left side is where all of the action happens. The left side is the powerhouse of the heart. It is the left atrium, which receives blood, that has been loaded with oxygen after passing through the lungs. This blood is forced into the left ventricle, which then gives the power stroke and forces this oxygen-rich blood out to the tissues of the body for use. Without the left ventricle, you are in big trouble. You cannot get oxygen to the brain, heart, kidneys, and other vital organs. The left, as I've stated, is where a great deal of the action happens.

This is not to suggest that the right side of the heart is unimportant. Oh no, you cannot have one without the other. The right side of the heart is the yang to the left's yin; balance is what the heart is all about. The squeezing of the right atrium occurs at the same time as that of the left atrium. The right atrium receives blood that has been depleted of oxygen after the tissues of the body have finished with it, then deposits blood into the right ventricle. From there, this blood, which is very low in oxygen, is forced to the lungs to pick up more oxygen. The blood then returns back to the left atrium full of oxygen and begins the round trip out to the body's tissues once again.

The heart, as a pump, is responsible for the perfect cycle of oxygen delivery to the body. Of course, there are many other aspects of the heart that describe and inform its function. There is an electrical system. There are valves located in between the atria and ventricles, as well as between the ventricles and the vessels into which they force blood. The heart muscle itself is a complex system in which form dictates function. But at its core, the heart is a pump, truly two small and two large pumps, made out of muscle. It is as essential an organ as an organ can be. It is so amazing that even outside of the body, unhitched from its vessels, it can "work" for some period of time because of the nature of the heart muscle fiber itself. The heart has what is called automaticity— it will stimulate itself for a period of time. Truly, this is a masterpiece designed by God, and although we can mimic it, we have not yet been able to match it.

The heart has its own unique electrical system that sets the timing of the beats of the heart. This system is complex and has built-in redundancy so that if one area fails, the heart will continue to beat. Oftentimes these default settings for rate control are not optimal for long-term (or even short-term, in some cases) function, but they may just buy enough time for intervention.

The problem with the heart is that its function can be altered by one little thing going wrong. A valve that has become inefficient, for example, may change pressures in one or more chambers, causing the heart muscle to grow as it adapts to perform harder (to overcome the new load). This muscle growth can reduce the overall function of the heart as a pump. As the output of blood is reduced and the normal quantity of blood is no longer going forward, it is forced to go in the only direction available. It backs up into the body's tissues, typically the lower legs or lungs (depending on which ventricles are involved). One domino falling causes more to fall, and the effects of these small failures over time are devastating on the heart and other body systems. It is for this reason that I emphasize repeatedly in this book that communication of new or concerning symptoms is the key to not just optimum function, but to survival in many instances. By informing your family and doctor of the discomfort you may have today, you may be identifying the first straw long before it breaks the camel's back. Please keep your loved ones and health professionals informed, as timing is everything with respect to intervention.

In the following chapters, we will look deeper into risk factors, disease states, and how the heart fails. Later, we will examine the effects of diet, exercise, and aging on the heart. It is my hope that you will look back at this brief description of the heart's function to help you better understand the heart and to help you appreciate the roles of some of the various parts of the heart. While in its purest form the heart is the perfect pump, we must remember that a lifetime of even the tiniest insults can disrupt its ability to work as intended. Remember these key aspects of living a long, healthy life:

Early and consistent education leads to prevention.

Early and quality communication leads to appropriate intervention.

Intervention increases the likelihood of survival.

CHAPTER 6
THE HEART ATTACKERS:
RISK FACTORS FOR
HEART DISEASE

"Doctor, Why?"

That simple two-word question is one that I get all too often and quite frankly is what motivated me to write this book. I usually get this question from patients at the beginning of a conversation about their diagnosis and treatment plan. In my case, as a heart surgeon, the focus of this conversation is usually centered on the need for bypass surgery or some other heart procedure. What is most notable to me is how often I hear this question asked.

Early on in my career, I was at times a bit perplexed as to why most people really did not seem to understand the nature of coronary artery disease or why it happened to them. I would frequently get the proverbial rhetoric, "I eat right and exercise. I never smoked," or, "We only eat fruits and vegetables and never any fried foods." Patients would tell me, "I take my medicines religiously," and without necessarily verbalizing it, what each patient was really trying to say to me was, in their own way, "Doctor, why me?"

As I've stated, this reaction was puzzling to me at that early stage in my career. Today, I welcome the question whether asked literally or inferred. The door has been flung open for me and I walk right in with my Heart Disease 101 lecture on the causes and treatment of heart disease. This is my chance to educate and communicate on the subject that I have become so passionate about.

Looking back at myself as a younger man and physician, I thought that most people would or should know more about what seemed to me to be common sense. Also, there was some degree of initial annoyance with patients when I heard questions that appeared to arise out of deliberate ignorance. As I've grown and seasoned, I've since realized that it is not deliberate ignorance that drives these questions. It is not necessarily even a lack of information or access to information that makes one ask "Why me?" when news turns out to be bad. It is a uniquely human trait that drives this sentiment: denial, that great defense mechanism that insulates each one of us. Denial is also one of several recurrent themes that drives decisions made by the individuals whose stories appear in this book. Denial begins with that first chest pain or the slow loss of function as a person notices they can't climb the same number of stairs as quickly as they used to. It begins when the heartburn troubling them continues in spite of incessant antacid use to keep down the pain. We all, intuitively, have the same sneaking suspicion that something is wrong but share the hope that "it's nothing." As I've stated several times and will continue to reiterate, communication, even of the most seemingly insignificant sign or symptom, is essential. Communication is all-important.

The Importance of Risk Factors— The Heart Attackers

Keeping in mind what I've said about denial, no single risk factor for heart disease can be ignored, nor does the development of coronary artery disease require multiple risk factors. In fact, there are cases where no known risk factor can be identified—a little troubling when you consider how unfortunate one must be to have no risk factors and still develop heart disease.

Although we know that our environment and diet are significant contributing factors, most people with heart disease have distinct risk factors that can be identified, and most importantly, managed effectively with a little commitment.

As we discussed earlier, anything that affects one aspect of the heart will cause a ripple effect that could eventually cause a problem with overall heart function. And while some of these problems with the heart are beyond our control (genetic issues, for example), the importance of managing risk factors that are known contributors to heart disease cannot be overstated. Imagine the heart as a pump that is in the bottom of a boat working hard to keep up with water that is spraying topside during a heavy storm. In this setting it would not be prudent to remove a wire or two, pour thick oil into the well in which the pump sits, or bang the pump with a hammer simply to see if it could continue to function. Perhaps the analogy is not perfect, but the point is clear . . . the heart is an amazing machine in which each aspect is interdependent.

The Risk Factors

Since the most common form of heart disease that directly affects the blood vessels is coronary artery disease, the risk factors we discuss here are mostly responsible for the development of this particular entity. However, as you progress through the book you will begin to see how many of the risk factors are interrelated and treating or managing one could benefit or reduce the impact of another. One example of this interrelatedness is exercise, which has been shown to reduce blood pressure, cholesterol, blood sugar, and help maintain a healthy body weight. Losing weight will lower blood pressure, cholesterol, and blood sugar. By adding an exercise regimen, not only are multiple risk factors affected positively, but specific risk factors (weight loss) will have additive effects on the same risk factors that exercise improves.

Risk factors fall in two categories. The first category is those risk factors that you cannot control, also known as nonmodifiable risk factors. These include:

- Age
- Gender
- Family history
- Race or ethnicity

We can't change the fact that we are getting older. Even if a man had a sex change, it would not reduce his relative risk of developing heart disease when compared to women. And women . . . you are not, unfortunately, off the hook. Remember Chapter 2: The Heart of a Woman! In fact, more women than men have heart attacks, and the death rate for women with heart disease is greater than that of men. Minorities are also at an increased risk for CVD—African Americans, Hispanics, and Native Americans are at particularly increased risk as compared to Caucasians. The fact is that although our genetic heritage may place each one of us at various degrees of risk, we all must be aware of what these are and minimize these risk factors that put us individually or collectively at risk.

How exactly do these nonmodifiable risk factors contribute to the development of heart disease?

Age
As we get older, our blood vessels get stiffer. They have had the cumulative effect of wear and tear as age and years of transporting large amounts of blood take their toll. It's quite remarkable to think that a person's heart beats sixty to a hundred times per minute every day for years—for their entire life. Imagine how much blood has been pumped through the arteries and veins of an eighty-year-old. And amazingly so, some have no evidence of atherosclerotic plaque buildup. Still, age reduces elasticity in certain key body tissues such as the blood vessels. This loss of give and take in the vessel walls translates into the heart (as a pump) working harder to move blood around the body.

Gender
Men have an increased risk of developing heart disease at a much earlier age than women. Men with multiple risk factors, including a family history, may develop heart disease in their forties and fifties. Men also tend to engage in unhealthy behaviors such as smoking, for example. The evil of nicotine is the effect that it has on blood vessels, constricting them and diminishing blood

to the heart via the coronary arteries. This reduction in blood flow to the principle muscle (the heart) that is busy providing oxygen to the rest of the body is a recipe for disaster.

With respect to women, while they may certainly develop heart disease in their forties or fifties, the incidence is very low. This differential between younger men and women is thought to be influenced by the protective effect of estrogen in women prior to menopause.

Family History

A person's family history is one of the most overlooked and underestimated risk factors among the "heart attackers," the importance of which cannot be overemphasized. We opened Part I of this book with a much deeper look at the importance and impact of family history. Stay tuned and keep reading.

A family history of heart disease in a first degree relative in their fourth and fifth decade imparts an increased risk to relatives of that person. Other risk factors such as high blood pressure, diabetes, and obesity tend to have a higher prevalence in family members as well. Thus it is important to know the medical history of family members throughout as many generations as possible.

Race or Ethnicity

African Americans and other minorities are at increased risk largely due to a higher prevalence of major risk factors in these groups such as high blood pressure, obesity, and diabetes. There may also be other confounders of increased risk that have yet to be explained through gene mapping and DNA analysis. What we know with certainty is that the heart attackers (high blood pressure, obesity, and diabetes) are highly prevalent in this group. Targeting these risk factors as individuals as well as in a group may well improve these statistics.

The following are the risk factors that you can control and thus directly lessen their impact. These are the modifiable risk factors. They include:
- High blood pressure
- High cholesterol

- Obesity
- Diabetes
- Lack of exercise
- Smoking
- Stress

High Blood Pressure

How does high blood pressure cause coronary artery disease?

Longstanding elevated blood pressure causes significant changes to the inner lining of blood vessels. These blood vessels then become more susceptible to the damaging effect of other known risk factors including elevated cholesterol and diabetes. Elevated blood pressure also increases the work of the heart. The heart has to expend more energy with each heartbeat in order to move blood out into the vascular system. Over time, this leads to changes in the heart muscle called hypertrophy, which is a thickening of the wall of the heart. Hypertrophy is a result of the heart muscle working harder to pump blood. This overcompensation will ultimately lead to heart dysfunction and heart failure.

What is a normal blood pressure?

While we're on the topic, you may ask yourself, what is normal blood pressure? Normal blood pressure should be somewhere around 120/80. The top number is called the systolic blood pressure and is created by the squeezing or contraction of the heart muscle. The bottom number is called the diastolic blood pressure and is created by the relaxation of the heart muscle. The systolic blood pressure in older persons will be higher due to the stiffening of the walls of blood vessels with age. Both numbers are important. However, the diastolic (or bottom number) is the number that determines the degree of high blood pressure in most people. In other words, we physicians worry more about the diastolic pressure in patients as a general rule.

When should I take my blood pressure?

It is an excellent idea to take and record your blood pressure first thing in the morning before beginning any physical activity, and certainly before that morning cup o' joe. Sit down and relax awhile and take your blood pressure with any number of commercially available automated devices. You can pick one up at your local drugstore. It is also a good idea to take your blood pressure at various times throughout the day, especially in the days following any changes to medications or when you have just been diagnosed and are beginning treatment.

Don't forget to keep a record of the trend as well. It is important to know at what times blood pressure is elevated or normal in order to properly adjust medications. Some over-the-counter devices save the prior readings so if you forget to write it down, the machine may have a record of it. Modern-day technology such as cell phones, tablets, and watches contain many different ways to record your pressure so that you can add it to your record when you get home. A record of this kind will be very informative to your physician. They can note trends and possibly gain insight into reasons for individual readings. I repeat—communication is the key to optimal health.

Can my high blood pressure be cured?

Unless your high blood pressure is related to a secondary cause, such as some forms of hormone-producing tumors or other surgically correctable causes, it is incurable. In particular, heart surgery will not cure your high blood pressure nor will it negate the need for your blood pressure medications. However, blood pressure can be controlled with a good medical regimen including exercise, lower salt intake, weight loss, and antihypertensive me-dications. So, while there is no known cure for high blood pressure, management is possible.

High Cholesterol

Contrary to popular thinking, cholesterol is necessary for normal bodily functions. It plays an important role in the makeup of cell walls and in the production of hormones. The problem with cholesterol is not necessarily cholesterol itself, but its imbalance created by improper nutrition and in some cases heredity. Most of this imbalance in cholesterol metabolism is created by a diet rich in saturated fats. The liver makes most of the circulating cholesterol and the remainder is supplied by our diets. When this process is not in balance the results can be devastating.

How does cholesterol cause heart disease?

There are several different types of cholesterol. These include high density lipoprotein (HDL), which is considered good; low density lipoprotein (LDL), which is bad; and triglycerides, which are bad if increased in the bloodstream. Technically speaking, triglycerides are not cholesterol, but are a lipid and have similar negative effects on the body when found in high-enough levels in the blood.

- HDL is a major transport substance that is made up of mostly protein. It helps remove cholesterol from the walls of arteries and takes it to the liver for processing and removal.

- LDL is involved in transporting cholesterol particles away from the liver and plays a major role in the development of atherosclerotic plaques within the lining of blood vessels. The plaque-developing characteristic of LDL is the reason for its well-deserved bad reputation. Plaque not only stiffens the blood vessels, which in turn raises overall blood pressure, but if broken free from the lining of a vessel, it poses serious risk to tissue downstream. Free-floating solid material (plaque) can obstruct a vessel partially or completely, creating a situation where tissues in the heart, lungs, brain, etc. that depend upon oxygen delivery are deprived of that oxygen. The results can be fatal.

- Triglycerides as a lipid (fat) are the result of regularly eating more calories than are burned. When this occurs, triglycerides are stored in the fat cells for later use (burned for energy). High levels of triglycerides in the bloodstream are thought to contribute to atherosclerosis and at very high levels may cause acute pancreatitis.

What are normal levels of cholesterol?

Total blood cholesterol<200
HDL cholesterol>50
LDL cholesterol<130
Triglycerides<150

While these are the typical normal levels of cholesterol, if you have other risk factors including high blood pressure, diabetes, smoking, and prior heart problems, then your health-care provider may recommend LDL levels less than 100 to minimize your exposure to risk.

Do I have to take medicines to control my cholesterol?

Medications called statins play an important role in the management of cholesterol imbalances. However, these medications are even more effective when you exercise, avoid high-fat foods, and lose weight. Although they may be necessary in a number of instances, you may be able to achieve lower doses when combined with exercise and proper nutrition. As I've mentioned, these risk factors are all interrelated, as are the treatments to reducing risk factors. Exercise, diet, and weight loss are a great place to start fixing many of these issues.

Are there any other ways to control cholesterol?

Yes, in fact, more and more evidence is being reported on the beneficial effects of omega-3 and omega-6 fatty acids. These are found in high concentrations in fish and certain plants such as flaxseed. They can play an important role in balancing the deleterious effect of LDL cholesterol.

In addition to the fish oils, soluble fiber may help to lower cholesterol. Soluble fiber is found in large quantities in fruits and vegetables and in even higher concentrations in some over-the-counter fiber products.

The Obesity Epidemic

According to the Centers for Disease Control, over 60 percent of Americans are either overweight (BMI>25) or obese (BMI>30). And even more disturbing is the growing problem of obesity in children. An estimated 16 percent of kids are obese [14]. Of course, this may be understated if you consider the difficulty of measuring obesity in children who are still in a growth phase. Nevertheless, the problem is well-documented.

Body mass index is the contemporary measure of weight. It is the weight in kilograms indexed to the height in meters squared. There is no factor in this calculation for the "big-boned" or "large-framed" person, so BMI may need to be adjusted in individuals who are not of an average frame. Still, BMI is the best way to estimate one's body fat composition and is widely used today.

How does obesity contribute to the development of heart disease?

The potential consequences of obesity—hypertension, diabetes, and high cholesterol—are thought to increase the risk of heart disease. There has been some research done on the "overworked" heart theory that may be a factor in the super obese. The main thrust of this theory is that the heart works overtime to supply blood flow to fat as well as the other "normal" cells that require oxygen provided by the blood supply. All of this extra work over a span of time would be harmful to the heart, according to this theory. While this seems plausible, the applicability of this theory is much less clear in the usual scenario of the overweight and obese.

Obesity is also the main driver of the epidemic of type 2 diabetes because it leads to insulin resistance, which is the precursor of type 2 diabetes. This fact leads us to our next heart attacker.

The Diabetes Epidemic

Diabetes is a major risk factor for heart disease. This is obvious when you consider that most (75 percent) diabetics succumb to heart disease. And as we outlined above, obesity seems to be the driver of the diabetes epidemic in the US. Once again, notice how these risk factors are interrelated. Estimates are that over 25 million Americans are diabetic—16 million diagnosed and another 8 to 10 million undiagnosed (realistically closer to 15 to 20 million undiagnosed) [15].

The majority of diabetics are type 2. Type 2 diabetics may have adequate circulating insulin levels, but their body's cells do not respond to insulin appropriately, leading to an increase in blood-sugar levels. Type 2 diabetics do not necessarily require insulin injections to control their blood-sugar levels. In fact, blood-sugar levels in type 2 diabetics can be controlled with diet and exercise alone if done appropriately.

Type 1 diabetes affects approximately 10 percent of diabetic patients. The problem in type 1 diabetes is a lack of insulin production in the pancreas. Most type 1 diabetics require supplemental insulin injections to control blood-sugar levels.

How would I know if I am diabetic?

Some common symptoms of increased blood-sugar levels include: fatigue, frequent urination, excessive thirst, and weight loss, which is ironic since obesity is considered a risk factor for the development of diabetes. If symptoms suggest diabetes, then a simple blood-sugar test will likely show elevated. Further confirmation can be done by administering a glucose challenge test. This may not be necessary in most cases, as a persistently elevated blood-sugar in the right context is sometimes all that is required.

The hemoglobin A1C is also a useful test to monitor long-term (three-to-four-month) control of blood glucose levels or a lack thereof. This is an important test to monitor treatment in known diabetics. The level should be less than six in most cases. This suggests better glucose control over time and implies a lower risk of developing complications related to diabetes, including heart disease.

How does diabetes cause heart disease?

A complex question, but here is what we do know. Diabetics have high blood-sugar levels; this is called hyperglycemia. As is the case of other heart disease risk factors, hyperglycemia contributes to the injury of the lining of blood vessels. The response to this injury is called inflammation. In cases where there are multiple risk factors in play, the atherosclerotic (hardening) process begins much earlier than in those cases where there are fewer risk factors. Thus, diabetes not only induces injury, but the hyperglycemia associated with diabetes contributes directly to the dysfunction of blood vessels and the development of atherosclerotic plaques.

Lack of Exercise

Depending upon what you read, this risk factor may be referred to as "physical inactivity." This implies that "physical activity" of any kind is acceptable, and that, unfortunately, is just not the case. Therefore, I like the term "lack of exercise," which means activity that is directed at increasing cardiovascular performance.

People who engage in regular physical exercise are much less likely to develop heart disease, primarily because they tend to have lower blood pressure, a lower BMI, lower cholesterol, and fewer instances of diabetes. In my observation, they also tend to smoke less and feel less stressed. Get it? Exercise lowers the impact of all of the risk factors for developing heart disease.

How much is enough?

The current recommendation of exercise for maintaining a minimum level of fitness is thirty minutes a day, six days a week. But it's not just the time that you put in that matters. It is also what you do in the time that you put in that counts.

I am often asked, "How far should I walk or run?" Well, that depends upon your level of fitness and any other physical limitations that may impede your ability to exercise. A good rule of thumb is to maintain your target heart rate for at least thirty minutes, six days a week. The target heart rate is 220 minus your age. This can be reduced by a factor of 0.85 in women or in those with physical limitations. The formula for women or individuals meeting the physical limitation criteria would be 220 − age × 0.85.

What if I don't have time?

I think most of us have time, but what we lack is commitment. We are consistently inconsistent. The good news is that you don't have to do it all at once. You can break up the routine and do it at ten to fifteen minute intervals, or if you prefer, you can do longer sessions fewer days of the week.

If you really think about it, it is not much time. Three hours out of 168 hours in a week is not much to ask when you consider that each hour of exercise may add an additional hour to your life expectancy [13]. Now I would say that is a pretty solid investment with a 100 percent return. If you really like numbers, then three hours is less than 2 percent of the available time in a week. That is a great investment!

Smoking

Smoking of any kind is a major risk factor for heart disease. It is estimated that up to 25 percent of heart attacks are directly related to the effects of smoking. In particular, women who take birth control pills and smoke have an even greater risk of all types of heart disease than their age-matched counterparts. Nicotine in the cigarette smoke, along with a number of other chemicals, causes direct damage to the lining of blood vessels and constriction of these vessels that leads to decreased blood flow. These chemicals also increase the work of the heart by increasing the heart rate.

Signs, Symptoms, and Diagnosis

What's the difference between a symptom and a sign?

Symptoms are what you feel and are usually what will send you to the doctor, like palpitations, chest pain, or fatigue. Signs are those things that can be evaluated by physical exam, such as: wheezing, leg swelling, irregular heart sounds, or abnormal diagnostic testing.

So how does it feel to have an ailing heart?

Before I answer that question, let's explore the issue in general terms. The classic symptoms of heart disease vary depending upon the underlying problem. For example, women have different symptoms than men in the face or absence of (or with or without) diabetes. Frequently, diabetics do not feel chest discomfort in the manner that nondiabetics might. It is extremely important to remember that in a majority of people with coronary artery disease, the first indication of trouble is a heart attack. This is true in over 50 percent of men and over 60 percent of women. That is not to say that they had no symptoms, but they did not recognize the symptom as an indication of heart disease. Particularly, men will describe episodes of "heartburn" or indigestion. Women will often refer to vague symptoms such as fatigue, palpitations, or anxiety. I call these instances the "asymptomatic paradox," because with very careful, detailed questioning these are in fact likely symptoms of heart disease, but not realized as such. Now just how would I know that? Because in my experience, the vast majority of people with severe disease treated with stenting or bypass surgery report an improvement in those not-so-troubling symptoms that were present prior to the intervention.

The most dramatic and disturbing symptom is chest pain, also called angina. This, like many signs of heart disease, is not a diagnosis. It has to be diagnosed. In plain English: you need to know why you are experiencing chest pain.

Patients with chest pain may describe it as a burning or stabbing sensation in their chest. Occasionally, the discomfort is described as chest heaviness or pressure. Pain that originates as a result of a heart problem may be felt in the jaw, neck, shoulders, or arms, particularly the left arm. This is called referred pain and is related to the remnants of nerve connections that were present when the body was developing as a fetus.

Shortness of breath, also called dyspnea, may or may not occur with chest pain and may be the only indication of a heart problem. Shortness of breath is thought to be a symptom of a dysfunctional heart's inability to meet the physical demands of the body. For instance, walking up a flight of stairs may initiate the sensation of shortness of breath or difficulty breathing.

Other symptoms may include: an irregular heartbeat or palpitations called an arrhythmia that may be felt as a sudden racing of the heart, anxiety, fatigue, generalized weakness, sweating, or diaphoresis and heartburn. Some signs of heart disease include leg or abdominal swelling, an irregular pulse, a heart murmur or extra/abnormal heart sounds, and wheezing.

The Symptom Conundrum

This all sounds great, but unfortunately, the first sign or indication of a problem with the heart is in the setting of a heart attack. As previously stated, this is particularly true for women who oftentimes do not manifest the classic signs of heart disease. This fact highlights the importance of being in tune with your body, understanding those subtle symptoms that could indicate a heart problem, and then communicating these experiences.

On the other hand, in my experience over the past twenty years I have noted that men have a much greater tendency to have "heartburn" or symptoms similar to gastro-esophageal reflux (GERD) disease, mimicking true heart pain. I have cured many a patient of GERD with a good bypass operation.

How do you know you have it?

Understanding the risk and symptoms are first. Regular visits to a health-care provider will help you identify and understand your risk of developing heart disease. Next, a good history and physical examination by a health-care provider may identify risk factors and physical findings that may indicate a heart problem. In particular, those persons with risk factors may need further testing to identify risk factors that may play a role in the development of heart disease. These include body mass index, blood pressure, cholesterol, blood sugar, and hemoglobin A1C in diabetics.

Remember, the details that help your health-care provider arrive at an appropriate diagnosis start with you, the patient. It is the recognition of signs and symptoms on the patient's part that become the difference between early intervention and the alternative. To illustrate the point, it is easy to diagnose heart difficulty when a patient is in the cardiac cath lab and fluoroscopy clearly shows that a blockage of a major vessel is the responsible factor for a heart attack. My work is more challenging when a patient presents to me mild heartburn or a vague sense of pain in the back. When patients present this information to me early (when first experiencing these symptoms), I am much more likely to arrive at a solution that will result in early intervention, typically resulting in much more favorable outcomes. The bottom line here is to communicate, and then, just when on the verge of becoming a royal pain, communicate some more. You are your own best advocate.

Chapter 7
The Heart-a-Tactics:
The Consequences
of Heart Disease

Heart Attack-Myocardial Infarction
Every forty-three seconds, someone suffers from a heart attack ... [2]

How to Navigate This Chapter
This chapter is designed to guide the reader through general heart-related knowledge, addressing specific disease-related questions and medications specific to treating heart disease. It is certainly helpful to read the chapter completely through to enhance understanding, but the chapter may also be used as a glossary to gain knowledge of specific diseases or conditions of interest.

Everything You Need to Know about the Heart

What is a heart attack?

A heart attack or myocardial infarction is caused by coronary artery disease that involves the buildup of atherosclerotic plaques within the lumen of the blood vessels of the heart. In general, these plaques develop slowly over years. Buildup of this plaque can lead to small heart attacks that often go unrecognized, chest pain (angina), irregular heartbeat (arrhythmia), and/or heart failure.

In the most dramatic cases, plaques rupture and lead to an abrupt interruption of coronary artery blood flow. If not properly treated in a timely fashion, this can lead to cardiac arrest and death. The most important steps you can take to lower your risk of developing heart disease are identifying and modifying risk factors through proper nutrition, regular physical activity, and avoidance of risky behaviors such as smoking and excessive alcohol consumption.

What are the warning signs of a potential problem with my heart?

First and foremost, you must recognize that you are at risk and then take steps to modify those risk factors which pertain to you. Recall that risk factors may be nonmodifiable (gender, race, family history, etc.) and modifiable (elevated blood pressure, diabetes, etc.). Recognizing the risk factors for heart disease is the first step toward reducing their impact on health.

Secondly, visit your doctor regularly, take an honest personal assessment of your health status, and ask lots of questions. Preparing a list of questions before your visit is a practical way to stay focused on achieving thorough communication of your experiences. You might also bring along any charts that you've created that trend blood pressure, blood sugar, or weight loss/gain.

Next, you must understand the **symptoms** that may signal a problem with the heart. Understanding these symptoms and their seriousness will help you recognize them should they occur.

How is heart disease diagnosed?

The diagnosis of a heart attack begins with recognizing the signs, symptoms, and risk factors. It starts with a good physical examination, health history, and risk assessment. Blood cholesterol and glucose levels are also checked when appropriate. Blood pressure should be checked. There are also several blood tests that can be performed to assess signs of heart muscle damage if a heart attack is suspected.

Beyond the basic laboratory assessment, several other noninvasive procedures may be recommended by your doctor in order to gain a more detailed understanding of what is happening. These might include:

- Chest x-ray
- EKG
- Echocardiogram
- Stress test
- CAT scan

If coronary artery disease is suspected after noninvasive testing is performed, then a heart catheterization is done to take a closer look inside the lining of the coronary arteries. This coronary catheterization provides the roadmap for the performance of a bypass operation should one be necessary or helpful.

How is heart disease treated?

In the setting of a heart attack, the best outcomes are achieved by immediate medical attention. Time is muscle, especially heart muscle. Depending upon the condition of the victim, immediate treatment may require something as simple as supportive care with oxygen, IV fluids, and pain medications, or at the other extreme, emergency bypass surgery. These decisions are best made by trained medical personnel and thus victims must seek medical attention immediately.

The most important thing to prevent a heart attack is to understand your risk factors and make good lifestyle choices, which include good nutrition and daily exercise. However, once the diagnosis is made, risk factor modification and medications are the foundation for any treatment plan.

Do I need to take medicines?

Yes. Most people need to take at least three heart medicines every day. Doctors can prescribe a wide variety of different types of heart medicines. The medications you take will depend on your heart condition and how your heart attack was treated. Some heart medicines help prevent chest pain and other heart symptoms. Other heart medicines help prevent future heart attacks and help you live longer. To prevent another heart attack, you will probably need to take aspirin and possibly another medicine every day.

If you have high blood pressure, high cholesterol, or diabetes (high blood sugar), your doctor will likely prescribe medicines to treat those conditions as well, since these are risk factors for heart disease (or the worsening of heart disease). Having untreated high blood pressure, high cholesterol, or diabetes can increase your chance of having another heart attack.

Your doctor might also tell you to avoid certain medicines, like nonsteroidal anti-inflammatory drugs (NSAIDs), for example. NSAIDs include ibuprofen (sample brand names: Advil, Motrin) and naproxen (sample brand name: Aleve). The use of NSAIDs in patients with heart disease actually worsen the condition, so pay close attention to medications that your doctor suggests you avoid.

It is also important to take your medicines exactly the way your doctor prescribes them. Let your doctor or nurse know if you have previously had any side effects or problems with the medicines. You should also let him or her know if you can't afford your medicines. There are often ways to solve these problems; free samples are often given out by drug reps and your doctor may be able to offer these to you.

What are the medications used to treat heart disease?

Some medications are directed at the underlying risk factors, including:

- Antihypertensives for **high blood pressure**
- Statins to **lower blood cholesterol**
- Hypoglycemic agents to **lower blood sugar** in diabetics

Others may be used to treat the symptoms of heart disease:

- Beta blockers to **lower the heart rate**
- Nitroglycerin for **chest pain**
- Diuretics to control **edema and swelling**

Special Considerations with the Use of Medications

Remember, all drugs have side effects! These are not necessarily allergies as some might think. True allergic reactions are characterized by swelling, difficulty breathing, rashes, itching, and in the most severe cases, low blood pressure, cardiovascular collapse, and potentially death. Most minor side effects tend to ease off the longer you take the medication causing the side effect. Others may persist and require discontinuation of the drug, switching to another agent in the same class, or switching to a new class of drug altogether.

It is important to distinguish side effects from true allergies for two reasons: first, true allergy could lead to severe consequences as described above. Second, one might be inclined to avoid a particular medication because of a minor side effect when, in fact, the benefit of a drug outweighs the annoyance of a minor side effect. This may prevent you from taking advantage of a potentially life-saving benefit. It is always a good idea to take this into consideration and talk to your caregiver.

Another important aspect of managing your medications is understanding interactions with other drugs whether prescribed, over-the-counter (OTC), or supplements. Always inform your pharmacist and caregiver of **all** medications and health or nutritional supplements you are taking. Doing so could save your life.

For clarity, drugs are often listed in publications and advertisements by their trade name, i.e., the brand name designated by the manufacturing company. This is followed in parentheses by the generic name, which is the name that is given to the chemical compound and is universally accepted. You will usually see it written like this: Trade (generic name). Therefore, some drugs with different trade names are actually chemically the same or very similar. For consistency, pharmacies usually label drugs by their generic name.

Please note: For a detailed description of medications used to treat heart disease, please see the appendix.

What happens after a heart attack?

After a heart attack, also called a myocardial infarction or MI, your doctor will make a treatment plan with you. The goal of this plan is to prevent another heart attack and lower your chance of dying from heart disease.

Do I need to make lifestyle changes?

You might. After a heart attack, your doctor or nurse will talk with you about:

- **Quitting smoking** – If you smoke, quitting smoking can lower your chance of getting or dying from heart disease. To stop smoking, some people find it helpful to:
  - Use nicotine patches, gum, or nasal sprays instead of cigarettes (nicotine is the main drug found in cigarettes)
  - Work with a counselor to find ways to make it easier to quit
  - Take a prescription medicine to reduce cigarette cravings
- **Getting exercise** – Getting regular exercise can keep your heart healthy. Your doctor or nurse will suggest an exercise program that is safe for you. Most doctors recommend that people exercise thirty to sixty minutes a day, five or more days of the week. In your exercise program, you should include three main types of exercise:
  - "Aerobic exercise" to raise your heart rate (examples of aerobic exercise include walking, swimming, and jogging)
  - "Resistance training" to make your muscles stronger (you can use weights or exercise bands to do these exercises)

- Stretching your muscles and joints
- **Improving your diet** – Eating the right foods can help keep your heart healthy. Fruits, vegetables, and foods with fiber can help prevent heart disease and strokes. Try to avoid eating foods that can make heart disease worse. These include "trans" fats, which are found in many fast foods, and "saturated" fats, which are found in red meats and many cheeses.

If you are overweight, it's important to lose weight. Losing extra weight lowers your chance of having another heart attack.

What is cardiac rehab?

"Cardiac rehab" is short for "cardiac rehabilitation." It is a special type of care people receive after having a heart attack. In your cardiac rehab program, doctors, nurses, and other health professionals will teach you how to keep your heart healthy. This includes ways to:

- Exercise safely
- Improve your diet, stop smoking, and control your other health conditions
- Cope with feeling sad or worried after your heart attack

When can I have sex again?

Having sex during the first two weeks after a heart attack could lead to more heart trouble. Check with your doctor about when it is safe to start having sex again. The timing will depend on the size of your heart attack, if you had problems after your heart attack, and if you still have symptoms.

After a heart attack, some people are less interested in sex or do not enjoy sex as much. This can be caused by certain heart medicines. This condition can also happen if people are worried about having a heart attack during sex. If you have problems with sex, let your doctor or nurse know. He or she might be able to treat those problems. Once more, communication is the key.

When can I drive again and return to work?

Check with your doctor about when it is safe for you to drive again and return to work. Most people can drive again one week after their heart attack. Many people can return to work within two weeks of having a heart attack.

What symptoms should I watch for after I've had a heart attack?

After you have a heart attack, you should watch for chest pain or symptoms of another heart attack [16]. People who have a heart attack have a higher than normal chance of having another heart attack and other heart problems. If you think you might be having another heart attack, **call for an ambulance right away (in the US and Canada, dial 911)**. Also, do not try to get to the hospital on your own.

Conditions Affecting the Heart

Listed below are conditions and problems associated with the heart and heart disease. These explanations contain information that is meant to serve as a resource for those affected by or wishing to understand heart disease and its related conditions.

Coronary Artery Disease

What is coronary artery disease?

Coronary artery disease (CAD) involves the buildup of atherosclerotic plaques within the lumen of the blood vessels of the heart. This can lead to several problems including chest pain (also called angina), heart attacks (or myocardial infarction), palpitations (or arrhythmias), and heart failure.

How will coronary artery disease affect me?

The risk factors, which include those that are not modifiable (that you **CANNOT** control) are:

- Family history
- Age
- Gender
- Ethnicity

And the modifiable (that you **CAN** control) risk factors:

- Smoking
- Diabetes
- High blood pressure
- High blood cholesterol
- Physical inactivity
- Lack of exercise
- Overweight
- Obesity
- High-fat diet

Identifying and modifying risk factors through proper nutrition, regular physical activity, and avoidance of risky behaviors such as smoking and excessive alcohol consumption are the most important steps you can take to lower your risk of developing heart disease.

Heart Valve Disease

Heart valve disease encompasses those conditions that lead to the malfunction of one or more heart valves. The heart needs these valves so that it can function as a blood pump. There are four valves separating the four chambers of the heart.

Diagram of the Heart Valves.[1]

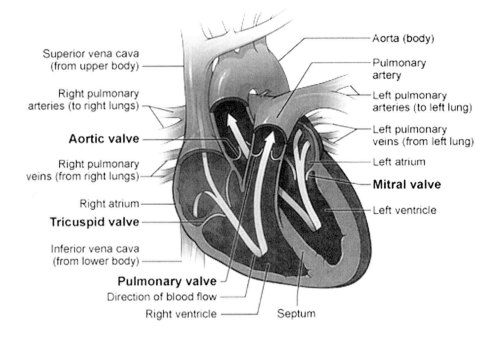

Aorta (body)

Superior vena cava
(from upper body)

Pulmonary
artery

Right pulmonary
arteries (to right lungs)

Left pulmonary
arteries (to left lung)

Aortic valve

Left pulmonary
veins (from left lung)

Right pulmonary
veins (from right lungs)

Left atrium

Mitral valve

Right atrium

Left ventricle

Tricuspid valve

Inferior vena cava
(from lower body)

Pulmonary valve

Direction of blood flow

Right ventricle   Septum

In the order that blood flows through the heart, these valves are:

1. Tricuspid
2. Pulmonic
3. Mitral
4. Aortic

So what are the heart valves and what do they do?

The heart valves function as one-way valves that allow blood to go through but not return to the heart chamber from which it originated.

---

[1] "Heart Valve Disease," University of California San Francisco Department of Surgery, accessed March 28, 2016,
http://www.pediatricct.surgery.ucsf.edu/conditions--procedures/heart-valve-disease.aspx.

With each heartbeat, blood leaves the upper chambers (the atria) and moves into the lower chambers (the ventricles). On the right side of the heart, the tricuspid valve separates the right atrium from the right ventricle. On the left side, the mitral valve separates the left atrium from the left ventricle. After a short delay, the heart beats again, forcing blood from the ventricles. On the right side, blood traverses the pulmonic valve and goes into the lungs. On the left side, blood leaves the left ventricle, crosses the aortic valve, and is received by the aorta—the largest blood vessel in the body. This continuous circuit leads to the "pumping" action of the heart muscle.

Although heart valve problems are a part of the spectrum of cardiovascular disease, they occur less frequently than other forms of cardiovascular disease. Heart valve diseases do occur more frequently in those people with risk factors for other forms of heart disease; in particular, those with high blood pressure and high blood cholesterol.

Dysfunction of heart valves usually manifests as regurgitation (a leaky valve that allows blood to flow backward) or stenosis (a blockage or narrowing that prevents blood from flowing smoothly across a heart valve).

There Are Two Categories of Heart Valve Disease:

1. **Congenital** – Individuals who are born with a valve problem, as in the case of a bicuspid aortic valve (should be tricuspid)
2. **Acquired**
   a. Age-related calcification in those over sixty-five
   b. Kidney failure causing calcification
   c. Idiopathic – unclear etiology
   d. Infectious – related to an infection on the heart valve; rheumatic fever
   e. Secondary – due to high blood pressure causing aortic valve dysfunction or heart attacks, leading to mitral valve regurgitation
   f. Mitral valve prolapse

What are the risk factors for heart valve disease?

The risk factors for heart valve disease include:

- Age
- IV drug abuse
- Procedures that require instrumentation of a body cavity or IV therapy
- Congenitally deformed valves (bicuspid aortic valve)
- Mitral valve prolapse
- History of infection of a heart valve (endocarditis)
- Family history of heart valve problems

What are the signs and symptoms of a heart valve problem?

The Signs and Symptoms of a Heart Valve Problem Include:

- Heart murmur – remember, this is not a diagnosis in and of itself, but it needs to be diagnosed
- Fatigue
- Shortness of breath
- Heart palpitations
- Leg swelling
- Chest pain

How Can I Detect a Heart Valve Problem?

Understanding risk factors is always the most important first step in the prevention, treatment, and recognition of any heart problem, and heart valve diseases are no different. In particular, if you have been told you have a heart murmur or a family history of heart valve problems or any other risk factors, then a trip to the doctor is always in order. Routine visits to the doctor will ensure that the problem does not go undetected for long periods, which otherwise may lead to irreversible heart failure.

How is the diagnosis made?

Diagnostic Tests for Heart Valve Problems Include:

- Chest x-ray
- EKG
- Echocardiogram
- Heart catheterization
- MRI

The most important test to diagnose heart valve problems is the echocardiogram (referred to as the "echo"). Echo utilizes ultrasound technology to bounce sound waves off of the internal structures of the heart, including the valves. When combined with pulse wave Doppler, the diagnosis of a specific valve problem is easily made.

The Echocardiogram Will Provide Important Information Regarding:

- Valve area – how wide or how narrow is the heart valve opening?
- Degree of regurgitation
- Degree of stenosis
- Heart chamber size
- Pumping function of the heart muscle

This information is extremely helpful in determining the need for valve surgery. Also of note, there are no lab tests for heart valve disease. Lab tests are used to assess one's overall risk of developing heart disease. So generally, diagnosis of valve problems is achieved with diagnostic testing.

What are the consequences of a dysfunctional heart valve?

- Chest pain
- Blackouts, a.k.a. syncope
- Palpitations, a.k.a. arrhythmias
- Sudden death
- Heart failure

How are heart valve problems treated?

Medical treatments for heart valve disease are directed at the underlying cause, if it is known. If there are risk factors for heart disease, then these are treated as indicated.

Medical Treatments May Include:

- Blood pressure medications
- Cholesterol-lowering drugs
- Drugs for chest pain
- Diuretics to treat swelling
- Nitroglycerin for chest pain
- Antibiotics in the case of valve infection
- Calcium control in kidney-failure patients
- Prophylactic antibiotics in the case of a known deformed valve such as mitral valve prolapse or bicuspid aortic valve
- Drugs to control palpitations

For those with a known heart valve problem, frequent follow-up and routine echocardiograms can detect progressive valve deterioration and subsequent failure. However, the most definitive form of treatment for heart valve dysfunction is surgical replacement or repair. Most aortic valves are replaced, and most mitral valves can be repaired depending upon the cause of the valve dysfunction. Surgery is generally reserved for the most severe forms of heart valve dysfunction when there are signs and symptoms of deterioration in heart function present.

Signs and Symptoms of Deterioration in Heart Function:

Aortic stenosis ("stiff" or "calcified" valve):

- Chest pain
- Syncope (passing out)
- Heart failure
- Severe stenosis (valve area < 1.0cm)
- High pressure gradient across the valve (>50 mmHg)

Aortic regurgitation ("leaky" heart valve):

- Chest pain
- Heart failure
- Severe regurgitation and enlarging heart chambers

Mitral stenosis ("stiff" or "blocked" valve):

- Heart failure
- Atrial fibrillation
- Transient ischemic attack (TIA) or mini stroke
- Severe stenosis (valve area < 2.0cm)
- High pressure gradient across the valve (>10mmHg)

Mitral regurgitation ("leaky" valve):

- Heart failure
- Severe regurgitation
- Atrial fibrillation

Milder forms of heart valve dysfunction may need to be treated when another type of open-heart surgery is planned, such as bypass surgery. This will allow a better short-term outcome and prevent the need for a second procedure in a short period of time, if the dysfunctional heart valve deteriorates further.

You may notice that I did not mention tricuspid or pulmonic valve procedures. This is because pulmonic valves rarely require treatment in adults, although they are commonly involved in congenital heart valve problems in children. Tricuspid valve dysfunction in adults is usually secondary to mitral valve dysfunction, infection, or heart failure and generally responds to treatment of the primary cause. Frequently, the tricuspid valve can be repaired at the time of mitral valve surgery. Infection of the tricuspid valve, called endocarditis, generally responds well to antibiotic therapy and rarely requires replacement or repair.

Atrial Fibrillation

So what is Atrial Fibrillation (AFib)?

Atrial fibrillation (known as AFib) is a common problem experienced by individuals in which the rhythm of the heart is abnormal. AFib must be treated; it is not a benign condition, as it increases the risk of stroke, heart attack, and other problems.

AFib is the result of the malfunction of the systems that control the heartbeat. In this condition, electrical signals that normally conduct the heartbeat along a predictable path begin to originate from locations other than the normal, expected location. This causes the top two heart chambers (the atria) to become unable to pump blood effectively, resulting in some blood being left behind after each stroke of the heart. This blood pools and is highly susceptible to forming clots, which can travel throughout the body to the brain, the heart itself, and other organs. It is for this reason that AFib is considered a serious condition, since these clots can cause stroke, heart attack, etc.

It is possible for AFib to be transient in patients (to appear and then go way without intervention). In many people, the condition becomes permanent, and when this happens, long-term strategies need to be implemented in order to decrease the risks associated with AFib.

What are the risk factors for AFib?

AFib has both nonmodifiable and modifiable risk factors, which are listed and described below. Please note that some of the modifiable risk factors that are listed are only considered modifiable if able to be controlled through treatment.

The Risk Factors for AFib Include:

Nonmodifiable Risk Factors

- Age (the older we become, the greater the risk of acquiring AFib)
- Heart disease (Congenital, coronary artery disease, congestive heart failure)
- Family history

Modifiable Risk Factors

- Obesity
- Heart disease (valve problems)
- Hypertension (if treated and controlled)
- Diabetes (if treated and controlled)
- Sleep apnea (if treated and controlled)
- Chronic kidney disease (if treated and controlled)
- Excessive alcohol use
-

What are the signs and symptoms of AFib?

The list below are signs and symptoms commonly reported by patients. Keep in mind that everyone is different, and your specific signs and symptoms may present differently. Report any concern you may have to your physician.

The Signs and Symptoms of AFib Include:

- Heart racing, skipping, or beating out of time is reported by many patients
- Mild pain or tightness in the chest
- A dizzy or lightheaded feeling
- Difficulty breathing

How can I detect AFib?

An EKG (also called ECG or electrocardiogram) is the most common test used to determine AFib. If you've never experienced this test, it is quite painless. This is a simple exam where leads are placed along your chest wall so that the physician can determine your hearts rhythm, rate, and any anomalies in the heart rhythm or electrical conductivity of the heart.

How is AFib treated?

AFib, once identified, can be treated with medications, cardioversion, ablation, pacemaker, and/or other surgical procedures. Medications are typically the first line of attack to treat AFib. Usually these medications consist of types that control the rate of the heart. Also, medications are used to keep clots from forming in blood, which may be more likely to occur in areas of the heart where blood is pooling during uncontrolled episodes of AFib.

Cardioversion is another method of treating AFib. This is a procedure performed in the hospital. While not a surgical procedure, you will receive medication to cause a sedative effect while a low current is sent through the heart. This current is necessary to attempt to "reset" the heart's rate and return it to its original rate.

In some cases, if other methods fail, it may be necessary to perform radiofrequency ablation. Also known as ablation, this treatment is essentially the directed use of heat or cold (cryoablation) to destroy the part of the heart sending the abnormal signals.

Pacemakers are also used to control AFib if the AFib is not responding to other treatment. A pacemaker will, as its name implies, directly set the pacing (or rate) of the heart to prevent the negative effects of AFib.

Abdominal Aortic Aneurysm and Thoracic Aortic Aneurysm

So what is an aneurysm?

Simply put, an aneurysm is a bulging of the walls of a vessel—in this case, the aorta. The aorta receives blood pumped directly from the left ventricle of the heart. This vessel is responsible for bringing oxygenated blood from the lungs to the entire body. As the vessel curves downward, it travels through the chest area and then the abdominal area. It is in these two regions, the thoracic and abdominal, that aneurysms often occur.

When bulging occurs in a person, there is a risk of rupture, as the wall of the vessel is weakened by the bulging caused by constant pressure. Consider the aorta (or any arterial blood vessel) as being like a garden hose. Under normal conditions, when water is turned on at the spout and the end of the hose is capped with a handheld sprayer, the hose is able to handle water pressure exerted on its inner walls. If, however, one were to compromise the wall of the hose by exposing it to high heat, for example, the hose would begin to bulge in that weakened area and potentially burst.

This example is similar to what is occurring in the heart. As pressure is exerted on the inner walls of the aorta, the wall may weaken over time if the pressure exerted is extremely high or if there is some other abnormality in the wall itself that has caused any weakening. This compromised area of the vessel then bulges, and when the "bulging" is greater than 50 percent of the expected diameter of the vessel, an aneurysm is said to exist. Keep in mind that what is normal for one individual may not be for another, as gender (males have, in general, larger-diameter vessels) and body habitus have an effect on "normal" size.

Classification of Aneurysms

Aneurysms are typed I through V according to their location within the body (not their size), Type I being higher up in the thoracic (chest) region and Type V much lower in the body. Aneurysms are also classified by their shape; fusiform aneurysms involve the entire circumference of the vessel, while saccular aneurysms are an outpouching of the vessel. Also, it is important to understand that aneurysms are not unique to the thoracic and abdominal regions of the body. They may also occur in the aortic arch (the first portion of the aorta where it is connected to the left ventricle of the heart) and other areas of the body.

What are the risk factors for an aneurysm?

The risk factors for an aortic or thoracic aneurysm include:

- Any risk factor for atherosclerosis: smoking, hypertension, high cholesterol, etc.
- A known aneurysm in the thoracic or abdominal aorta
- Certain diseases or disorders in which connective tissue is weakened as a result: Marfan's and Loey's-Dietz syndromes, for example.
- Aortic valve disease (bicuspid valve, aortic valve replacement, or stenosis [narrowing])
- Family history of aneurysm or dissection
- Cerebral aneurysm

What are the signs and symptoms of an aneurysm?

In the case of thoracic aortic aneurysm, there are usually no symptoms until the aneurysm has become so large that pain results.

The Signs and Symptoms
of an Aneurysm Include:

- Chest, back, flank, or abdominal pain
- Nerve dysfunction due to compression of nerves by the aneurysm
- Hoarseness, diaphragm paralysis, wheezing, coughing, or shortness of breath

How can I detect an aneurysm?

Since many patients do not experience pain until the aneurysm increases substantially in size, aneurysms are often discovered via a CT scan that has been ordered for some other condition. CT scan or MRI is a definitive method that your physician will use to diagnose an aneurysm.

What are the consequences of having an aneurysm?

Left untreated, the potential for rupture of the vessel may occur, which is a life-threatening situation that requires immediate emergency surgical intervention. If this occurs, the patient will experience severe pain and a rapid decrease in blood pressure. This is an EMERGENCY!

How are aneurysms treated?

Once symptomatic, surgical intervention is a must.

A Rare but Dangerous Bunch—
Patent Foramen Ovale-PFO

What is a patent foramen ovale?

A patent foramen ovale (PFO) is a small opening between the top two chambers of the heart (the right and left atrium). This opening allows blood to flow between the two chambers. This occurrence is actually normal in a fetus, but usually closes shortly after birth. However, in some cases the hole fails to close; a fairly common condition that occurs in one out of four people [17].

What are the signs and symptoms of a PFO?

There are no signs or symptoms that would be attributable to a PFO, only late signs or symptoms of stroke or other event. Please read below for more information.

What are the consequences of a having a PFO?

There is a rare but possible side effect of leaving a PFO untreated. If a blood clot were to happen in a leg, for example, and this were to travel to the heart, there is the potential that the clot could then cross the right atrium into the left atrium and then flow from the left ventricle somewhere into the brain or to another organ. This could cause a stroke or ischemic event (lack of oxygen) to the affected organ.

Is there a test for a PFO?

Using what is referred to as a bubble test during an echocardiogram (echo), a physician can get a clear picture of the heart in action. This allows visualization of blood flow.

How is a PFO treated?

If you have not had symptoms (related to stroke or other serious consequences), treatment of PFO is not necessary. If, however, you have had a stroke as the result of the PFO, you will likely be placed on an aspirin regime to prevent clotting and possibly be recommended surgery to close the hole.

Less invasive methods of helping to prevent blood clots are also recommended when you have been diagnosed with a PFO.

- Do not sit or stand still for long periods of time
- Walk around every one to two hours if you have been sitting still or on a long trip
- Change position when sitting, moving legs and feet occasionally
- Do not smoke

Atrial Septal Defect (ASD)

What is an Atrial Septal Defect?

ASD occurs at birth; it is a congenital condition and is the most common lesion in adults occurring in the aortic valves [18]. The aortic valve is the valve that controls blood flow from the left ventricle into the main systemic arteries (the arteries that supply fresh, oxygenated blood to the body). A lesion on the valve can create many problems with the heart, as well as other areas of the body, as is explained below.

What are the signs and symptoms of ASD?

Signs and symptoms are related to the effects of other problems caused by having ASD: pulmonary hypertension, right-sided heart failure, atrial arrhythmias (unusual heart rhythms and AFib, for example), blood clot formation, and brain abscesses (lesions in the brain). Symptoms appearing from these conditions are wide-ranging, complex, and often interrelated. Generally, any shortness of breath, chest pain or pressure, head pain, or persistent wet, nonproductive cough should be reported to your doctor.

How Is ASD Detected?

Echocardiography (echo) is the method that physicians choose to diagnose ASD. There are many types of echo procedures performed to aid in diagnosis. The transthoracic echo used together with a bubble study is one method. A two-dimensional echo is sometimes used to differentiate ASD. This method essentially allows for a more detailed picture that captures specific forms of the condition. A three-dimensional echo may also be used for extreme precision in diagnosing difficult cases.

CMR and CAT scan imaging is sometimes performed in patients, and although these provide valuable information, they are not considered the gold standard in diagnosing ASD due to the limit in technology.

Doppler imaging is sometimes used (again not representing the gold standard of assessment). There are limits to the value of this type of imaging since certain types of defects may be missed.

Cardiac catheterization is rare, since diagnosis can be achieved by noninvasive testing as described above.

What could happen if ASD is not treated?

The concerns with ASD are (as mentioned) right-sided heart failure, pulmonary hypertension, atrial arrhythmias, blood clot formation, and brain lesions. These are all serious and potentially life-threatening conditions that must be addressed.

Coronary Artery Abnormalities

What does having an abnormal coronary artery mean?

The coronary arteries supply oxygen-rich blood directly to the heart. The small arteries usually develop normally during the growth of the fetus, but occasionally do not. Oftentimes even without completely normal development there is no clinical impact (patients have no symptoms and heart function is completely within normal limits). There are several abnormalities though that, when they occur, can be quite detrimental to function, if not outright deadly.

Anomalous aortic origin of a coronary artery (AAOCA) is one congenital defect that is particularly dangerous. This occurs when the left main coronary artery or the left anterior descending artery originates from the right sinus or right coronary artery. Similarly, the right coronary artery originating from the left sinus or left anterior descending is also problematic. This abnormal positioning can cause the vessel to become compressed by other structures in the area leading to heart attack (MI) and sudden death. This is often seen in teenagers and adults alike.

What are the signs and symptoms of AAOCA?

Unfortunately, this congenital heart condition may not be noticed until death has occurred. Often, this is the cause of young athletes who suddenly die on the field without a warning to indicate any problems. Luckily, the likelihood of sudden death in patients with AAOCA is low.

The signs and symptoms of AAOCA (if they do manifest) include:

- Chest pain or pressure
- Myocardial infarction (MI)

How is AAOCA detected?

Coronary magnetic resonance angiography (CMRA) is an excellent way for your doctor to diagnose AAOCA. Coronary angiography by computed tomography is also a useful way to make the diagnosis and is noninvasive, unlike the CMRA. Also, coronary computed tomography angiography (CCTA) is a rarely used but helpful modality to diagnose this congenital disorder. Stress studies with echo or radionuclide myocardial perfusion imaging are another way of assessing the situation.

When is AAOCA treated?

Treatment of AAOCA is a complex matter, except in the case of patients who are symptomatic. In these patients, surgical intervention is a must. Typically, symptomatic patients experience arrhythmias of the ventricles, which are usually life-threatening, or they have had an MI. For patients in these circumstances, any risks that may be associated with surgery are far outweighed by the risks of not undergoing surgical intervention.

In asymptomatic patients, surgical intervention is often a debated point among physicians. At the least, consideration should be given to the patient's preference, age, overall vitality, and risk associated with surgery. Once these issues have been addressed, both the physician and the patient can make an educated decision that weighs out risk versus reward.

Other considerations as to whether or not to proceed to the surgical suite in asymptomatic patients may be swayed toward intervention when exercise-induced ischemia (blood flow reduction to the heart during exercise) is present in a patient.

How is AAOCA treated?

Surgical intervention used in patients with AAOCO include coronary artery bypass grafting (CABG). Alternatively, stents may be placed to help avoid the complications of ischemia for those patients experiencing it.

Congenital Conditions That Are Associated with AAOCA:

- **Tetralogy of Fallot** – This is a congenital condition in which approximately 5 to 15 percent of patients with the condition have a single coronary artery [19].
- **Transposition of the great arteries** – These patients typically have a wide variety of coronary artery anomalies. Typically, the right coronary artery (RCA) and the left main coronary artery originate from areas where they should not due to abnormal development of the arteries during fetal development.
- **Truncus arteriosus** – Rarely, patients with this condition may have coronary arteries that are located over the anterior portion of the right ventricle. When this occurs in a patient, the possibility of injury to this vessel during surgical procedures becomes a serious risk.
- **Bland-White-Garland syndrome** – Coronary and other arteries that supply blood to the heart originate from the pulmonary artery, which may result in ischemia, leading to heart failure in these patients.

Coronary Artery Stenosis

Coronary arteries may become narrow (stenotic) for various reasons: they may not be fully developed or may be dilated and, thus, subject to aneurysm. These conditions may sometimes require surgical intervention to correct them.

What is coronary artery narrowing?

Narrow (stenotic) coronary arteries can be congenital or acquired. Acquired stenosis of the coronary artery may be caused by Kawasaki disease, familial hyperlipidemia, or certain drugs, e.g., methysergide, prior to surgery that has altered the vessel. Syphilis and Takayasu arteritis are other diseases that may have been acquired in a patient and are known to cause stenosis.

Narrowing due to a congenital condition may occur when the coronary artery is positioned in such a way as to become compressed by another structure during fetal development. Williams syndrome is one such congenital disorder in which the location of the coronary arteries causes enlargement of the inner portion of the artery, which in turn narrows the artery.

What are the risks of having a narrow or stenotic coronary artery?

Living with a stenotic coronary artery means that blood supply to the heart is compromised. As a result, flow is less than it ought to be, meaning that oxygen supply is also minimized. This can cause chronic pain (angina) in the chest area and lead to myocardial infarction (MI)—**heart attack**.

What are the risk factors for developing a coronary artery stenosis?

- Hyperlipidemia (elevated cholesterol and triglycerides)
- Hypertension
- Prior cardiac surgery
- Congenital or acquired disorders of the coronary artery (as previously described)

What diagnostic tests are used in patients with coronary artery narrowing?

For patients with risk factors for stenosis, long-term surveillance is recommended to determine the need for intervention. This surveillance takes the form of imaging (noninvasive or invasive angiography). Assessment for ischemia (again, lack of blood flow) caused by the stenotic coronary artery is done through stress testing (either exercise or pharmacologic) and/or with noninvasive imaging (echo or nuclear imaging).

How is coronary artery stenosis treated?

If testing determines that surgical intervention is necessary, patients can expect to undergo CABG or epicardial laser revascularization. Percutaneous coronary intervention (PCI) using stents (or not, depending upon findings) is also another option to improve blood flow to the heart due to a narrow coronary artery.

Coronary Artery Enlargement

Coronary artery enlargement is also either congenital or acquired. Acquired enlargement occurs when an enlarged ventricle operates under increased demand or due to a small connection (fistula) between the coronary artery and the pulmonary artery. Patients who acquire this condition usually suffer from a disease that involves the coronary arteries like Kawasaki, for example.

Coronary Artery Aneurysm

Coronary artery aneurysm (ectasia) describes an artery in which a segment is dilated. This may be due to congenital conditions such as connective tissue diseases (polycystic kidney disease, Ehlers-Danlos syndrome) or from a number of acquired conditions or diseases. Atheromatous disease, Kawasaki disease, syphilis, Takayasu arteritis, trauma, dissection, angioplasty, or atherectomy are all potential causes of coronary aneurysm.

What are the complications of
having a coronary artery aneurysm?

The prime complication that is most concerning is rupture and/or thrombosis. Rupture is rare but could happen because of the weakened vessel wall, which is constantly under pressure; recall the comparison of an artery to a garden hose. Thrombosis may occur due to slow blood flow in the immediate area of the aneurysm. A blood clot could travel directly to the myocardium (the heart muscle itself), causing ischemia.

How is a coronary aneurysm evaluated and treated?

Evaluation is done by a resting and stress radionuclide myocardial perfusion imaging test. This exam uses thallium, which enables assessment of the adequacy of perfusion to the myocardium and its overall function. Coronary angiography is done to assess the size of the aneurysm and to determine which treatment options are appropriate. Treatment may ultimately involve resecting the aneurysm, followed by a CABG.

Coronary Artery Fistulae

Coronary artery fistulae are essentially a connection between vessels or other areas of the heart that should not be connected (a coronary artery to a heart chamber, for example). These are usually due to congenital defects, although they may be acquired with trauma (gunshot, stab wound, etc.) or during invasive procedures involving the heart (pacemaker implantation, biopsy of the myocardium, or angiography).

These atypical connections between vessels or chambers of the heart can cause problems with blood being rerouted to an area of the heart other than the intended area, which may cause excess blood in that area, bringing with it an entire new set of problems.

What are the symptoms of a coronary artery fistula?

If small, blood flow to the heart will not be affected enough to produce symptoms. However, if some of the blood intended to go to the myocardium (the heart muscle) is lost to another area because of the fistula, ischemia will result. Ischemia, you will recall, is the lack of blood flow resulting in less oxygen delivered to tissue, which typically results in chest pain.

Some Symptoms of Coronary Artery Fistula Include:

- Chronic angina
- Pulmonary hypertension
- Heart failure
- Myocardial infarction (MI)
- Endocarditis
- Heart rhythm abnormalities
- Thrombosis or aneurysm
- Rupture of the fistula (rare)

How is a coronary artery fistula diagnosed?

Often, a murmur can be heard by a physician upon examination. The murmur is loud and continuous. X-ray and EKG may show a coronary artery fistula if the fistula is large enough. Ideally, an echo (two-dimensional) can make the definitive diagnosis. CAT scan is another method sometimes used to diagnose coronary artery fistula. To further identify size and features of the fistula, coronary angiography may be used.

How is a coronary artery fistula treated?

If asymptomatic, there is generally no need to treat. If, however, fistulae are large, a ligation is performed to close it. In the case of small fistula, your doctor may suggest closing it electively (even without symptoms) since these tend to get larger with age. This choice is usually made when there is a murmur present that concerns your physician.

Closure of fistula are frequently performed during a cardiac catheterization, although percutaneous techniques have been used with good results.

Persistent Sinusoids

Similar to coronary fistulae, persistent sinusoids create a link between cardiac chambers and coronary arteries. Yet instead of this connection happening because of a fistula, it occurs due to a capillary that connects the two. These are congenital in nature.

How are persistent sinusoids diagnosed?

Doppler echo is used if there is enough blood flow to capture an image useful enough for the physician. However, persistent sinusoids are more often diagnosed with angiography.

Final Thoughts

While there are many causes of heart disease, there exists a bottom line to the path that untreated heart disease takes. Left untreated, in most patients, there is a predictable result—the overall failure of the heart to function as designed. The heart is the perfect pump. It has been structured to disperse blood throughout every artery in the circulatory system of the body, depositing oxygen-rich blood to tissues. Without this pump operating at its full potential, patients experience a wide range of signs and symptoms (from minor irritations to death). With recognition of these signs and symptoms and a healthy approach to minimizing risk factors, every one of us increases our chances of living longer and healthier lives.

CHAPTER 8
THE FAILING HEART

Heart failure is a condition that occurs when the heart cannot pump or fill with enough blood, which means that the heart must work harder to deliver blood to the body's tissues. The term "heart failure" is misleading because the heart does not completely fail or stop. Instead, the heart "fails" to do its most important function—to pump blood forward. As a result, blood begins to pool in the veins that supply the heart with the blood that it must pump. This pooling of blood causes swelling, typically in the legs (ankles usually bear the brunt of this and may appear swollen and dark purple in patients who have suffered from multiple severe attacks). The edema caused in the lower extremities can cause skin issues, a heavy sensation in the legs, and wounds caused by cracking skin. Sometimes blood can back up so much that fluid is forced into the lungs, which can cause very serious symptoms.

As you can see, there are various degrees of heart failure, from mild to severe with accompanying symptoms that range widely. Thankfully, although heart failure is a serious condition, there are safe and effective treatments available. Treatment can help you to feel better and live longer.

Types of Heart Failure Simplified

The heart is comprised of four chambers: the two upper chambers are the right and left atria, and the two lower chambers are the right and left ventricles. The left ventricle plays a key role because it pumps blood to the entire body. This ventricle is normally the strongest and is the chamber from which blood pumps out with the most force. Failure to pump can occur on the left side of the heart; this is called left-sided heart failure, and it may also happen on the right side of the heart, called—you guessed it—right-sided heart failure. Congestive heart failure is an umbrella term that encompasses both left- and right-sided heart failure. For example, a person suffering from right-sided heart failure in an acute exacerbation (worsening of signs and symptoms) would be said to be "in congestive heart failure." Let's look a bit more deeply at each type of heart failure.

Left-Sided Heart Failure

This type of heart failure happens when the left ventricle, the chamber in the heart responsible for moving oxygen-rich blood that has just come from the lungs, is not functioning properly. When the left ventricle's ability to pump is compromised, the heart muscle in this area must work harder to pump the same amount of blood. Over time, all of this hard work has consequences for the overall function of the left ventricle, and the heart muscle itself becomes progressively less functional.

There are two types of left-sided heart failure (systolic and diastolic failure), and drug treatments are different for each type. Systolic failure occurs when the left ventricle cannot contract in the normal way, making the force of each contraction weaker than it would normally be. Diastolic failure is what occurs when the heart muscle becomes stiff (the left ventricle in this case). Due to its stiffness, the left ventricle can't fill with blood properly during diastole (the period of time when the ventricle is relaxed—not contracting).

As blood builds up "behind" the pump, so to speak, if the pressure and volume of blood is great enough, blood can be forced through pulmonary capillaries and into the lungs. It is possible for this to happen on a nearly imperceptible scale, the patient unaware of what is occurring except for minor symptoms. But, as left-sided heart failure worsens over time, it can progress to the point of causing a wet-sounding but usually nonproductive cough, wheezing, and severe shortness of breath. These symptoms should be taken very seriously and a medical provider should be contacted immediately.

Right-Sided Heart Failure

While the focus of the left ventricle is moving oxygenated blood forward to organs and tissues of the body, the right ventricle is receiving this oxygen-spent blood after it has travelled through large veins that empty into the right atrium. This deoxygenated blood is then pumped back to the lungs for the drive-by oxygen pickup system that occurs there.

The function of the right ventricle is very much dependent on that of the left. If left-sided failure occurs, the increased pressure over time damages the right side. This is because of the systemic backup of blood transferring fluid pressure over to the right ventricle. Stated another way, the right ventricle must work harder to pump blood to lungs that are stiffer because of blood that has backed up due to a failing left ventricle. As you can see, the circulatory system is a closed system where any malfunction is felt in another part of the system.

When blood backs up as a result of failure of the right ventricle, it exerts pressure on the veins that are normally in the process of returning blood to the heart. These veins swell, and fluid pressure transfers some fluid to the body's tissues: legs and feet swell (edema), ankles swell, and ascites may occur (the liver is overwhelmed with fluid). In the lower extremities, this edema can become so severe that skin will crack and split because of the pressure. These signs take a fair amount of time to develop, so there is usually time for proactive treatment.

Congestive Heart Failure

Congestive heart failure is the end result of untreated heart failure or of the heart simply becoming overworked, and it requires timely medical attention. Sometimes congestive heart failure and heart failure are used interchangeably; however, technically speaking, heart failure implies a slow, chronic progression in which the heart is not functioning at par. Congestive failure refers to the acute worsening of signs and symptoms to the point where immediate medical attention is required.

This is exactly how congestive heart failure occurs: as blood flow out of the heart becomes less efficient, blood returning to the heart through the veins backs up, causing congestion in the body's tissues. Often, swelling (edema) results. Most often there's swelling in the legs and ankles, but it can happen in other parts of the body, too. Sometimes fluid collects in the lungs and interferes with breathing, causing shortness of breath, especially when a person is lying down. This is called pulmonary edema and if left untreated can lead to respiratory distress. At this juncture, the kidneys may become involved as their ability to rid the body of sodium and water is decreased, adding to the edema of body tissues and organs. Left untreated, death is likely to occur.

Heart Failure Causes

There are many causes of heart failure. Fortunately, with early identification and treatment, it is often possible to prevent or significantly delay the development of heart failure.

The common causes of heart failure are:

High blood pressure (hypertension): Due to the increased pressure in the arteries, the ventricles of the heart must work above normal capacity to offset the ever-present pressure. Over time, the heart muscle itself enlarges (similar to the way any other muscle in the body would enlarge as a reaction to increased work). Unfortunately, the enlarged heart muscle is not functionally sound and begins to lose the ability to pump blood forward as efficiently as it should.

Coronary heart disease: The coronary arteries normally deliver fresh, oxygen-rich blood to the heart, but when narrowed (stenotic), the heart muscle can become deprived of oxygen. Deprivation is noticeable in individuals during exercise (even light exercise, if the lack of oxygen is severe enough) as reduced exercise tolerance. Left untreated, this condition can progress to heart attack, as tissues are completely deprived of oxygen. Tissue that cannot be saved following a heart attack contributes to the overall weakness of the heart and further impairs function.

Heart valve disease: A number of conditions, including heart attack and aging, can damage the heart valves.

- Heart valves may narrow, causing interference with blood flow and increasing pressures that the ventricles must adapt to (leading again to an enlarged ventricle that is reduced in function).
- Valves can also become leaky. When this happens, the valve is termed an "insufficient valve." If the leak is severe enough, blood flows backward (regurgitation), adding to pressures that the ventricles must overcome to move blood forward. All of these issues, if untreated, lead to failure of the heart.
- It is possible for a valve to become both narrowed and leaky, adding insult to injury.

Cardiomyopathy: As the heart sustains increasing damage caused by insults to the heart muscle, its walls become enlarged, thick, and rigid—cardiomyopathy is the term used to describe the end result of this process. As you might imagine, this changing of the shape of the heart directly alters its function. Not only is forward blood volume reduced as muscle contraction force is reduced, but the electrical activity that controls heart rate and rhythm is affected, producing irregular heartbeats (arrhythmias). Congestive heart failure is sure to follow.

Symptoms of Heart Failure

As the amount of blood pumped by the heart (the cardiac output) decreases, a variety of signs and symptoms can develop. These are:

- Weakness, lightheadedness, or dizziness
- Shortness of breath
- Elevated heart rate (even at rest)
- Swelling in the lower legs and feet (edema) or in the abdomen (ascites)
- Feeling fatigued

Diagnosing Heart Failure

A medical history, thorough exam, and various lab tests are all used by physicians to determine heart failure. Here are some of the most commonly used:

- **Electrocardiogram (EKG)**: The electrical activity of the heart and specifically the path that the current takes can be clearly seen on an EKG, providing a "picture" of the heart's electrical activity. When things go wrong with the heart that alter this normal electrical path, the EKG can identify or at least point the way toward where in the heart the problem is occurring. Heart rhythm and rate are also easily assessed with the use of an EKG. The physician uses this information to see what is happening with your heart and where to focus medical attention.
- There is a **blood test** used to identify heart failure that identifies a protein (brain natriuretic peptide—BNP) that presents in an abnormally high concentration during heart failure. The test has many names: BNPT, N-terminal pro-BNP (NT-proBNP), and so on.
- **Chest x-ray**: An enlarged heart will show up on x-ray; recall that this sign is due to the heart having to work harder over a period of time to pump blood against

resistance. Also, during an acute heart failure episode, an x-ray will clearly display fluid buildup in the lungs, as this is a common sign during congestive heart failure.

- **Echocardiogram**: An echocardiogram, or echo, uses ultrasound (high-frequency sound waves) to assess the heart's size and valve function. Echocardiograms may be taken at different points in time and compared to assess changes in function over time.

- **Exercise testing**: Coronary arteries that are stenotic or blocked will reveal themselves during an exercise test known as a "stress test." By examining an EKG, your blood pressure, and heart rate at different points of time during the test, a physician can determine how your heart is tolerating exercise. Specifically, the EKG in this setting provides a "picture" of the function of the heart as exercise severity is increased throughout the testing period. An exercise test ("stress test") determines how well your heart performs during exercise. In this way, weaknesses caused by blocked or narrowed arteries may be identified. If these problems are found and are severe enough, there will likely be a need for further testing to pinpoint their exact locations.

- **Heart (cardiac) catheterization**: Cardiac catheterization helps to measure how well the heart is functioning, providing detailed pictures of the coronary arteries. During the test, a thin tube (the catheter) is inserted through a large blood vessel in the groin (or arm) and advanced into the heart. A dye is injected into the catheter to view the arteries and the structure of the heart by x-ray. As blockages are identified, they may be simply noted, or dealt with during the exam, depending upon severity.

- **Other tests**: Cardiac catheterization is an invasive test that can have risks. Other tests, like computed tomography or magnetic resonance imaging, are sometimes used to look at the coronary arteries. This type of test is recommended only in specific situations.

Heart Failure Complications

Heart failure can cause symptoms and make you feel ill. If severe enough, it may cause dangerous or even life-threatening complications. The goal of treatments for heart failure is to reduce symptoms and the chance of developing complications. The most common complications include:

- A weakened and enlarged heart muscle (cardiomyopathy)
- Irregular heart rhythms (arrhythmias), which can lead to blood clots or stroke
- Heart attack

Heart Failure Treatment

The course of heart failure is typically long term, meaning it is a chronic condition with periods of flare-ups that may require immediate medical treatment and may also be life-threatening. While typically able to be treated, heart failure is not per se curable, unless the cause is something purely mechanical that can be replaced (for example, a valve). The disease is best treated by diet and lifestyle changes, medical regimens that support normal heart function, and sometimes a pacemaker or defibrillator as a protective measure in an effort to keep your heart functioning normally or to prevent serious complications.

Diet and Lifestyle Changes

Changes in diet and lifestyle are often recommended to treat heart failure. The most common recommendations include:

Lowering your salt and water intake

Salt, in the simplest of terms, pulls water toward it. When the concentration of salt is high in the blood (after eating a number of large high-salt meals, for example), water is pulled from various places in the body and goes toward where it is naturally attracted—salt. This process causes the blood volume to rise inside the blood vessels. This action, in turn, increases the overall pressure in those vessels. When this process is severe enough, the heart must now pump hard to move blood around the body because of the extra amount of blood and the higher resistance. Add to this picture a weakened heart, one that is enlarged and functioning abnormally at baseline, and you have a big problem on your hands as blood backs up into the body's tissues in the legs, ankles, feet, and lungs.

It is therefore critical that the amount of salt (sodium) in food is kept to a minimum. The exact amount of salt that you should take in ought to be discussed with your doctor. Fluid is on the other side of this equation, and the amount taken in needs to be regulated by individuals with heart failure. Two liters (sixty-six ounces) is a good daily maximum for most people, although this may vary depending on several factors. Have this discussion with your doctor to get specific fluid limits for your situation.

Monitoring weight

Establish a daily routine of weighing yourself at the same time on the same scale. Many people will do this in the morning every day before breakfast, for example. Try your best to keep the amount of clothing you are wearing (shoes, etc.) the same so that you get an accurate picture of the trend of your weight.

A two-pound weight gain in a day is potentially cause for some alarm. You will want to let your health-care professional know. Also, more than four pounds in one week may be a sign of fluid buildup in your body; be sure to notify a health-care professional in this case as well. Sudden weight loss may also be a sign of heart failure, so keep track of any changes and report them.

Keeping weight under control

Being overweight has many negative consequences. For your heart, being overweight means working harder to move blood around the body and to supply all of the cells of the body with oxygen. This is a huge amount of extra work that your heart must conform to. This extra strain might be the breaking point for a heart that is already overworked.

Stopping smoking

One effect of the nicotine that is contained in cigarettes is that it causes blood vessels to constrict (to get smaller). Think of the physics here: when a flexible pipe that has no leaks or holes for fluid to escape is made smaller, a pump working to move fluid through that pipe has to work harder to get the job done. Your heart functions exactly the same way. It gets very scary very quickly when you realize that the pipes (the coronary arteries) that supply the heart with oxygen-rich blood also constrict when affected by nicotine. In the presence of nicotine, the heart must pump harder to supply itself with blood! This is not a good thing if the heart is not functioning at full capacity. The situation is worsened considerably when these coronary arteries are stenotic (narrowed) or blocked, and then the effects of nicotine are added to an already small vessel. Please consider trying to quit smoking, as this is extremely important to your heart health.

Limiting alcohol use

I will not use this forum to rail about the many issues with alcohol, but suffice to say that large quantities are not good for your health in general. A good rule of thumb is one serving per day for women and two for men, a serving being roughly twelve ounces of beer or five ounces of wine [20]. Drinking too much alcohol is not good for your heart or your health in general. If your heart failure is related to excessive drinking, stop drinking alcohol completely.

Cardiac Rehab and Exercise

Since shortness of breath is a common symptom of heart failure, exercise can be an important way to combat this symptom. Light exercise most days of the week may help to prevent worsening symptoms. Keep in mind that an exercise routine should be organized under the care of your doctor.

Medications

Medicines are often used to treat heart failure symptoms; some medicines have even been proven to prolong life. It is very important to take these medicines on time every single day. If you cannot afford or have trouble taking your medicines, talk to your doctor or nurse.

Some of the most commonly prescribed medicines include:

- **Diuretics:** This type of medication, Lasix being a prime example, is used to treat heart failure by getting rid of the excess fluid that builds up in the legs and lungs. In patients who are chronically experiencing this buildup of fluid, diuretics can keep the buildup from becoming unmanageable, particularly in people who keep close control over their water and salt intake.
- **Angiotensin converting enzyme (ACE) inhibitor or angiotensin II receptor blockers (ARBs):** By widening blood vessels, these medications relieve some of the pressure on your heart, making it possible to pump with less effort. It should be noted that ACE inhibitors may cause a side effect that is very specific to this medication; the patient may experience a dry cough and, if so, can be switched to an ARB-type medication instead.

- **Beta blockers:** By slowing the heart rate down, beta blockers can help the heart beat more efficiently.
- **Blood thinner:** One way to reduce the amount of resistance that the heart has to pump against, and also a way of avoiding blood clots in people with irregular heart rhythms (such as AFib), is to use a "blood thinner." Warfarin, commonly called Coumadin and/or Aspirin, is a commonly used medication to accomplish these tasks.

Heart Rhythm Treatment

When patients suffer from heart failure, they are at risk for a life-threatening abnormality in the rhythm of the heart. Different from an arrhythmia, which starts in the atria, a ventricular rhythm (starting in the ventricles) can occur. When this happens, the heart may become unable to pump enough blood to sustain life. At this point the heart must have a shock delivered in hopes of returning it to its former, controlled state. This shock is known as defibrillation, and often times a physician will recommend placing a small device called a defibrillator surgically in the chest. When in place, a defibrillator can automatically detect and deliver a shock capable of reversing this type of abnormal life-threatening rhythm.

Sometimes people with heart failure develop another type of abnormality in the electrical system of the heart that causes the left ventricle to beat in an uncoordinated manner. This also decreases the efficiency of the heart and can lead to congestive heart failure. There is a special type of pacemaker capable of helping the heart keep up called cardiac resynchronization therapy (CRT), a.k.a. biventricular pacing, that can treat this heart problem. It is sometime necessary to combine a pacemaker and a defibrillator to deal with both of these heart problems.

Surgery or stenting

When a heart valve is the reason for heart failure, surgery can be an option. It is not uncommon to include bypass grafts of the coronary artery(s) at the same time if necessary while addressing a valve problem surgically. Stents may be placed inside of the coronary arteries to keep blood flowing freely if a blocked or narrowed artery is the culprit for heart failure.

Treatment for advanced heart failure

In severe cases of heart failure that do not respond to treatment, heart transplantation may be necessary. Unfortunately, there are many reasons why a person may not be an appropriate candidate for transplantation, so careful screening must be done with each patient. Also, there are a limited number of available organs for transplantation; people often must wait many months or even years before one may become available.

If you require a heart transplant and there are no immediate prospects, your doctor may recommend a left ventricular assist device. This device may also be used in lieu of a transplant. The device is placed inside of the chest to improve the flow of blood by helping the heart directly when it is weakened.

Living with Heart Failure

While it may be frightening to be diagnosed with heart failure, there are a number of things that you can do to improve your chances of managing the condition:

- Always take your medicines even when you feel better. Skipping doses may cause symptoms to return. Remember, your medications help prevent the disease from advancing; you must stay on them religiously to benefit from them.
- If you are experiencing side effects from your medication, let your doctor know. There may be similar medications that will accomplish the same thing, or perhaps your dose could be slightly adjusted so you do not experience the side effect.

- When you feel symptoms getting worse, seek help; call your doctor or health-care provider. If things become difficult, do not hesitate to call 911. Do so if the following symptoms occur:
  - Severe shortness of breath
  - Chest discomfort or pain lasting greater than fifteen minutes and not improving after rest or nitroglycerin
  - Fainting or passing out
- Call your doctor or nurse if you develop any of the following, which can be signs of worsening heart failure:
  - Increasing or new shortness of breath
  - New or worsened cough, especially if you are coughing up frothy or bloody material
  - Worsened swelling in your legs or ankles
  - Weight gain of two pounds (one kilogram) in one day or four pounds (two kilograms) in one week
  - Fast or irregular heartbeat

Heart failure is a serious concern. If left untreated, heart failure that is chronic and may be producing little or no symptoms can progress rapidly and bring with it severe signs and symptoms that must be treated immediately. Be aware of which symptoms to report and when to report them. Never hesitate to call your health-care provider if something "just doesn't seem right." Early reporting means early treatment. Also, keep in mind the preventative behaviors that you can use to improve your chances of not developing congestive heart failure. Be mindful of your diet, stay as fit as possible, and stick to your prescribed medication regimen. Doing so may save your life.

PART III
TRIUMPH

CHAPTER 9
PUT ME OUT OF
BUSINESS, PLEASE!

The positive effects of holding to a healthy and consistent nutrition and exercise regimen have been proven ad nauseam, and when you get right down to it, the logic of sticking to these regimens simply makes sense. Simply look around you at the natural world—animals, for example. Can you picture a female lioness lying on the Serengeti day after day, eating to her heart's content, her meals provided by another? I'm sure you cannot, as this is not reality. To survive, she must be at the ready at all times to procure food. Exercise, top physical conditioning, is a must for her survival. She must be lean and driven. So must we.

So why do we feel (I include myself at times) that we can do just fine sitting at home, barely moving except to pass the remote or reach for the next sandwich? We must face the fact that this type of behavior is simply unnatural. We are built to be strong, focused, and tenacious creatures. Our bodies must truly be treated like our temples. Not doing so has disastrous results.

So how does one turn around a lifetime of sedentary living and eating fatty, processed foods? I've explained the motivation for doing so in previous chapters; potentially avoiding heart disease is one prime motivator. But once and for all taking a step toward health . . . this is a tall order, particularly in the young, who are naturally inclined to believe that the detrimental effects of lifelong unhealthy habits will not be felt until far into the future, if ever.

My goal as a physician and as one who has endured great physical, mental, and psychological challenges is to inspire you to reach for these goals. Think about the following for a moment: we all experience great challenges. No one is spared this reality of life. The other, hopeful part of life is that we are all extended grace. By that, I mean that as individuals we can turn our behaviors around, trying new ones on for size. Grace is available to us regardless of where we are with our lives. The best advice that I can give to anyone attempting to change or improve their behaviors is this: if you fail in your efforts to reach your fitness or dietary goals, get up and try again. Persistence is the key to successful change. Keep trying. This is my pep talk, which I hope you will find useful on your pursuit of living a healthy lifestyle.

As you progress through this chapter, you will learn about both nutrition and exercise and why each are so important to your overall health. Take from this what you will, but please take from it.

Eating to Live—Nutrition Basics

What is nutrition?

For our purposes, adequate nutrition is the intake of substances that fully meet a patient's metabolic needs, providing the body with enough of the nutrients necessary for optimal function. With respect to the heart, nutrition is everything. It needs all of the supportive nutrition that it can get.

Consequences of inadequate and unbalanced nutrition

Why bother to balance nutritional intake? Here is why: Inadequate or unbalanced nutrition impairs the body's ability to develop and maintain ongoing processes. Growth and repair of skin, hair, muscle, bone, metabolic rate, and the immune system itself all rely heavily on sound nutrition to thrive. Mental health, energy levels, physical endurance—all of these are a direct result of following a good nutritional balance. We might say that adequate and balanced nutrition is the basis of good health.

Inadequate or malnutrition may take the form of overnutrition. One of the side effects of this is obesity. In 2013, the American Medical Association declared obesity a disease because being obese is correlated to predictable signs and symptoms common to many in this demographic group. Obesity is a serious concern.

Undernutrition typically affects the very young and the very old. However, there are unfortunately many examples of under-nutrition of all ages in parts of the world where food and other resources are either scarce or highly controlled by one group.

While malnutrition in any form (under- or overnutrition) may have many causes, one commonality, largely with respect to obesity, is the lack of education. Overcoming this educational disparity is a driving force that motivates me.

Dietary guidelines and standards

Every five years, the US Departments of Agriculture (USDA) and Health and Human Services (HHS) convene a fifteen-member panel to update the nation's dietary guidelines. The panel's stated mission is to identify foods and beverages that help individuals achieve and maintain a healthy weight, promote health, and prevent disease. The guidelines also serve as the foundation for national nutrition policies, such as school lunch programs and feeding programs for the elderly.

The 2015 dietary guidelines include a number of positive modifications. One modification addresses what was long thought of as an enemy of the heart—cholesterol, once linked to heart disease and heart attack. The advisory panel has decided to eliminate these warnings about dietary cholesterol, which for decades has been wrongfully blamed for causing heart disease, because there is no such link. According to the report, "cholesterol is not a nutrient of concern for overconsumption."

Until now, the guidelines have recommended limiting dietary cholesterol to three hundred milligrams (mg) per day, which amounts to about two eggs. It is important to note that high-cholesterol foods do not necessarily lead to high blood cholesterol. On the contrary, high blood cholesterol is a result of carbohydrate conversion to fat and abnormal metabolism of fats in the liver. Saturated fats are a more important exogenous fat source to avoid. Bottom line, low-fat, low-salt foods are best in the setting of heart disease.

Trans Fat and Sugar Are the Dietary Culprits That Cause Heart Disease

Should I make a bolder statement? How about this one—stop eating trans fats and sugar . . . now! To protect your heart health, you need to address your insulin and leptin resistance, which is the result of eating a diet too high in sugars and grains. To safely and effectively reverse insulin and leptin resistance, thereby lowering your heart disease risk, you need to:

- Avoid processed foods and other sources of refined sugar and processed fructose, as well as refined grains. Whole grains are also best avoided if you're insulin and leptin resistant.
- Focus your diet on whole foods, ideally organic, and replace the grain carbs with:
  - Large amounts of vegetables
  - Low to moderate amounts of high-quality protein (think organically raised, pastured animals)
  - As much high-quality healthy fat as you want (saturated and monosaturated from animal and tropical oil sources)

At the risk of preaching to my audience and losing some folks (a risk, by the way, that I am willing to take if it means reaching the largest number of people), I want everyone to understand that we are at the mercy of nature. I have not and do not expect to see in my lifetime a cupcake, Twinkie, french fries, or milkshake in the paws of the average African predator. If we want to live long, productive, and energetic lives that are less likely to wrap up with ten or so years of weakness, illness, and debilitation, then we must take care of ourselves. Now!

Other Notable Changes in the 2015 Dietary Guidelines

The 2015 guidelines are probably better than they've been in decades. Among the most notable changes is a partial turnaround on artificial sweeteners. While they say artificial sweeteners such as aspartame are probably okay in moderation, they should not be promoted for weight loss.

Artificial sweeteners should be removed from the market altogether due to their numerous health risks, but at least the current recommendation reflects the voluminous evidence showing that artificial sweeteners do NOT promote weight loss. On the contrary, they tend to promote weight gain and have been shown to worsen insulin resistance and metabolic disorders to a greater degree than refined sugar.

The 2015 guidelines also reflect the shift away from focusing on specific nutrients such as fat, carbs, or protein—which in the past have led to an ever-growing plethora of processed "functional" foods—toward a general focus on eating more whole foods. My only objection here is that they still do not consider the hazards of eating too many whole grains, which can exacerbate insulin and leptin resistance. That said, the panel does recommend limiting refined grains.

As for the panel's review of research into foods that help combat disease, vegetables and fruits are the only dietary elements found to be consistently helpful against every disease included in the review. One can only hope that this will sink in and eventually lead to much-needed changes in agricultural subsidies, which are currently geared entirely toward the manufacturing of disease-promoting processed foods that are high in added sugars.

The 2015 guidelines also break new ground by commenting on the environmental impact of our food choices. The panel notes that switching to a healthier diet higher in veggies, fruits, nuts, and legumes and lower in animal products could reduce greenhouse gas emissions and consume less resources such as water and energy.

Sources for Credible Nutrition Information

It is advantageous as a consumer to position yourself to gain as much knowledge as possible. Take the time to read up on and discuss with others the information that you find. You may hear people say the following: "There are so many studies out there— you can just as easily find one to discount the other, so who knows what's real?" While there is a grain of truth to this statement, be careful to avoid the temptation of allowing this logic to rule your good common sense. For example, one might find a study that states that coffee is generally healthy to consume and another equally reliable source that finds coffee consumption to be unhealthy. After reading two opposing studies, the cynic may say, "Well, I'll simply drink coffee because I want to. Who knows which study is right?" Acting in this way is short-sighted. Without further investigation, this person would be acting on impulse. Maybe the two studies had an entirely different focus, and each study's conclusions were true.

The point is that very few things in life are that black and white. There may be various truths that exist independently within each study, even if these truths appear to be slightly contradictory on their face. Trust your gut and investigate. Reliable resources for nutritional information include:

- Food and Nutrition Information Center
- Health.gov: 2015 Dietary Guidelines for Americans
- Healthfinder.gov
- American Heart Association
- WebMD
- The Mayo Clinic

- Office of Dietary Supplements (ODS)
- CDC's Division of Nutrition, Physical Activity and Obesity
- Academy of Nutrition and Dietetics
- Medline Plus (NIH)

Metabolism

Metabolism refers to all the chemical processes going on continuously inside your body that allow life and homeostasis (maintaining normal functioning in the body). These processes include those that break down nutrients from our food and those that build and repair our body. Building and repairing the body requires energy that ultimately comes from your food. The amount of energy, measured in kilojoules (kJ), that your body burns at any given time is directly affected by your metabolism. A high metabolism means large amounts of energy burned, and the reverse is also true.

If we eat and drink more kilojoules than we need for our metabolism and exercise, we store it mostly as fat. Most of the energy you expend each day is used to keep all the systems in your body functioning properly. This is out of your control. However, you can make metabolism work for you when you exercise, effectively turning the tables on weight gain. Couple exercise behavior with eating the proper amount of calories necessary to fuel your body without over- or underconsumption and you have the magic bullet.

How does metabolism differ among individuals and at various stages in life?

After age forty-five, the average individual loses around 10 percent of their muscle mass per decade [23]. This equates to losing about one-third to one-half a pound of muscle each year and also gaining that much in body fat. Because muscle mass burns a lot of calories compared to fat, the total number of calories needed goes down as well.

How Aging Impacts Metabolism

Many studies have been done to understand why people gain weight as they age, and the answer is clear—the change in body composition accounts for the vast majority of the decline in metabolism.

There is also a growing number of studies, however, that suggest that body composition does not account for all of the weight gain associated with the aging process. Decreases in the calories used by the body's organs, such as the heart and liver, also seem to occur as the body ages.

Physical activity plays a role in both body composition and metabolism during the aging process. Research shows that most individuals gradually reduce their level of physical activity as they age, which further reduces their number of calories needed to maintain weight. Less activity also means less use of the body's muscles, which contributes to the general decline in muscle mass and subsequent changes in body composition.

Overall, these age-related changes mean that the average fifty-year-old woman needs around three hundred to five hundred fewer calories per day than she did in her twenties to maintain the same body weight [23]. So for those who gain weight while aging, the reason is not necessarily eating more, but rather eating the same while needing fewer calories. It is for this reason that every one of us must gain an understanding of how our bodies change as we age, as well as what constitutes proper nutrition.

Other Determinants of Metabolic Rate

Gender

Males usually have a higher metabolic rate than females (of the same age) because males tend to have a higher proportion of lean body mass than females of the same age. Conversely, females tend to have a higher proportion of fat cells, and fat cells have a lower metabolic rate than lean muscle cells.

Pregnancy

Metabolic rate increases during pregnancy and lactation due to the high energy requirement of producing fetal tissues and then breast milk.

Increased food intake

Eating large amounts of food requires the digestive system to process more material, which therefore requires more energy. However, as food is the source of the body's energy, any resulting increase in metabolic rate is likely to be less than the increase in energy intake due to the additional consumption of food. Bottom line: eat what your body requires if you want to maintain a steady weight. Eating more does boost your metabolism, but the effect of this boost in minimized by the resulting excess energy turned into actual weight gain.

Increased secretion of certain hormones

The thyroid hormones triiodothyronine (T3) and thyroxine (T4) are the main regulators of metabolic rate. Metabolic rate increases when the quantity of these hormones in the blood increases. Some other hormones such as testosterone, insulin, and human growth hormone (HGH) can also increase the body's metabolic rate.

Increased physical exercise

Exercise requires and uses energy. Although BMR is energy expended at rest, exercise has both short-term effects (during the time of the exercise itself) and long-term effects (after and between exercise sessions). One of the longer-term effects of frequent physical exercise is an increase in metabolic rate. This increase in BMR is due to increased overall activity of the heart and vascular system, together with other body systems and tissues.

Environmental Conditions

Extremes of temperature

When body temperature increases above or decreases below its ideal range, mechanisms within the body act to reduce or raise its temperature to preserve health (and ultimately life, as prolonged elevated body temperature can destroy proteins within the body and prolonged depressed temperatures can cause cardiac arrhythmias, which can be fatal in both cases). The body's temperature regulation mechanisms require and use energy.

If these mechanisms are often or continuously active, metabolic rate increases to allow for such activity and corresponding use of energy even when the body is at rest. In general, the higher the body temperature, the higher the metabolic rate (hence, metabolic rate is higher when a person has a fever).

Stress and anxiety

Stress is sometimes thought of as an unpleasant combination of overwhelming worry, anxiety, fear, and the feelings of constraint and helplessness. Such emotions are associated with physical responses within the body that vary but may include increased heart rate or blood pressure, difficulty sleeping, nausea, abdominal discomfort, increased sweating, etc. To the extent that these involve caused (e.g., increased heart rate), cause (e.g., difficulty sleeping) or are by (e.g., nausea, abdominal issues) increased bodily function and thus increased use of energy, metabolic rate increases accordingly.

Adequate Calorie Intake

Women

Because women generally have a smaller frame and less lean body mass than men, they usually require fewer calories. The US Department of Agriculture recommends women consume 1,600 to 2,000 calories if they are sedentary; 1,800 to 2,200 calories if they're moderately active; and 2,000 to 2,400 calories per day if they are active [24].

Men

The amount of calories men require each day varies based on their age and activity level. Calorie recommendations decrease with age. The US Department of Agriculture recommends men consume 2,000 to 2,600 calories if they're sedentary; 2,200 to 2,800 calories if they're moderately active; and 2,400 to 3,200 calories per day if they are active [24].

Children

Toddlers between the ages of one and two need about 45 calories per pound of body weight each day, which usually translates into something in the range of 1,000 to 1,400 calories per day. Since children this age have relatively small stomachs, this should be split between three meals and two or three snacks.

Three-year-old children also need about 45 calories per pound of body weight, which is between 1,000 and 1,400 calories per day. However, four-year-old children aren't growing quite as quickly, so they only need about 41 calories per pound of body weight, or about 1,200 to 1,600 calories per day. Preschoolers can be quite picky and easily distracted, so it may take longer for them to eat and it may take a bit of coaxing to get them to eat a healthy mix of foods.

School-age children need about 1,200 to 2,200 calories per day. Children between the ages of five and six need 41 calories per pound of body weight, and those between seven and eleven need 32 calories per pound [24]. Don't worry too much about your child not eating enough, since children this age usually eat when they are hungry. Serve healthy foods and encourage your child not to eat too many calories if they start to gain extra weight.

Elderly

As described earlier, the elderly have a lower rate of metabolism than those in the younger population. All things being equal, we often gain weight as we age because our caloric requirements decrease. This is why it is necessary to cut short our caloric intake as we age. This is true unless you are very physically active. The more active you are, the more calories you can eat. If you are a female couch potato over age fifty, the National Institute of Health Senior Health website advises you should eat no more than 1,600 calories a day. Kick your activity level up to moderately active, and your calories can go up to 1,800. Walk the equivalent of three or more miles a day at a brisk clip, and you might be able to take in 2,000 to 2,200 calories a day without gaining weight. Men who generally have bigger frames and more muscle mass are allowed 2,000 to 2,200 for low activity; 2,200 to 2,400 for moderate activity; and 2,400 to 2,800 for the active lifestyle [25].

Components of a Healthy Diet

A healthy diet is one that contains all the nutritional elements in optimum concentration. There are many dietary ingredients, each having their own importance.

A balanced diet contains six key nutrient groups that are required in appropriate amounts for health. These groups are outlined below.

- Proteins are involved in growth, repair, and general maintenance of the body.
- Carbohydrates are usually the main energy source for the body.
- Lipids or fats are a rich source of energy. They are also key components of cell membranes and signalling molecules, and as a component of myelin, they insulate neurons (nerve cells).
- Vitamins are important in a range of biochemical reactions.

- Minerals are important in maintaining ionic balances and many biochemical reactions.
- Water is crucial to life. Metabolic reactions occur in an aqueous environment, and water acts as a solvent for other molecules to dissolve in.

Proteins

Proteins are molecules made of amino acids. They are coded by our genes and form the basis of living tissues. They also play a central role in biological processes. For example, proteins catalyse reactions in our bodies, transport molecules such as oxygen, keep us healthy as part of the immune system, and transmit messages from cell to cell.

There are many different types of proteins in our bodies. They all serve important roles in our growth, development, and everyday functioning. Here are some examples:

- Enzymes are proteins that facilitate biochemical reactions. For example, pepsin is a digestive enzyme in your stomach that helps to break down proteins in food.
- Antibodies are proteins produced by the immune system to help remove foreign substances and fight infections.
- DNA-associated proteins regulate chromosome structure during cell division and/or play a role in regulating gene expression (for example, histones and cohesin proteins).
- Contractile proteins are involved in muscle contraction and movement (for example, actin and myosin).
- Structural proteins provide support in our bodies (for example, the proteins in our connective tissues, such as collagen and elastin).
- Hormone proteins coordinate bodily functions. For example, insulin controls our blood-sugar concentration by regulating the uptake of glucose into cells.

- Transport proteins move molecules around our bodies. For example, hemoglobin transports oxygen through the blood.

Carbohydrates

In a similar way to protein being made up of amino acids, carbohydrates consist of building blocks called saccharides, or sugars. Glucose, a common example of the simplest type of sugar, is a monosaccharide, together with fructose, found in fruit. Two monosaccharides joined together are called disaccharides, the most common being sucrose, or "white cane sugar," as we know it. Another example of a disaccharide is lactose, found in milk. When large numbers of saccharides are joined together, they form polysaccharides and are found in the foods we commonly think of as "carbohydrates," e.g., bread, potatoes, and pasta.

Dietary fiber belongs to the carbohydrate group but is not digestible. Fiber has important roles in helping you feel full after a meal, adding bulk to stools and preventing constipation, and for gut health in general. Fiber can be found in plant-based foods such as whole grains, lentils, and fruit and vegetables.

Carbohydrates are the main providers of energy in our diet. Every body cell, including the brain, requires a constant supply of glucose as fuel, most of which is provided by the carbohydrates in food and drink. Most foods contain some carbohydrates, but foods containing the most include fruit, vegetables, bread, breakfast cereals, rice, pasta, legumes (chickpeas and lentils), milk, yogurt, and sugar.

Current recommendations are that 45 to 65 percent of an adult's energy intake comes from carbohydrates [26]. Eating at least six servings of bread and cereals (preferably whole grain, i.e., not refined) and five servings of fruit and vegetables each day will help you reach the recommended level.

Fats

Foods and drinks contain nutrients such as carbohydrates, proteins, fats, vitamins, and minerals. Some foods or drinks contain a large amount of a single nutrient. For example, a soft drink contains a large amount of sugar, and fried food contains a large amount of fat. The terms "fat" and "oil" are often used to mean the same thing.

Dietary fat (fat in foods and drinks) is important for many body processes. For example, it helps move some vitamins around the body and also helps with making hormones. There are different groups of dietary fat, and each of the groups can have a different effect on your blood cholesterol level. For this reason, it is recommended that you replace foods and drinks high in saturated and trans fat with alternatives that contain more polyunsaturated or monounsaturated fats.

Each gram of fat contains twice the kilojoules (energy) of carbohydrates or protein. Because of this, if you have foods and drinks with too much dietary fat, it can be difficult to maintain a healthy weight. As I've stated, fat is a necessary component of the diet. Balanced proportions of the types of fat as well as the amount of fat in a meal are both very important to consider when analyzing the value of a given meal. Meals with a small amount of fat not only enhance taste, but also help to keep you satisfied for longer. Throughout the day you should consume a wide range of everyday, healthy foods. By doing this, you will get the reasonable total amount of dietary fat, particularly polyunsaturated and mono-unsaturated fats, necessary to meet your daily requirements.

The two types of blood cholesterol are low density lipoprotein (LDL) cholesterol and high density lipoprotein (HDL) cholesterol. LDL is considered the "bad" cholesterol because it contributes to the narrowing of the arteries, which can lead to cardiovascular diseases (such as heart disease and stroke). HDL cholesterol is considered to be the "good" cholesterol because it actually carries cholesterol from the blood back to the liver where it is broken down, reducing the risk of cardiovascular disease. An easy way to distinguish which cholesterol is good and which is bad is to remember the following: LDL stands for *lethal* density lipoprotein, while HDL can be thought of as *helpful* density lipoprotein.

Omega-3

Whether taken in supplement forms (pills, powder, etc.) or by eating fish, omega-3 may lower total cholesterol and triglyceride levels in the blood. Anything that can lower these levels is a good thing when considering heart-disease prevention or improving overall health. Remember that high levels of cholesterol and triglycerides are associated with increased risks for blood clots, stroke, and heart failure.

How much and what kind of fish do you need to eat? Basically, we're talking about two servings (3.5 oz) of fish, twice weekly. Also, salmon, trout, sardines, herring, and tuna are your best options.

The benefits of omega-3 fatty acids include:

- lower triglyceride levels and reduce blood pressure, which are important risk
- factors in cardiovascular disease
- improve blood vessel elasticity
- keep the heart rhythm beating normally
- "thin" the blood, which makes it less sticky and less likely to clot
- reduce inflammation and support the immune system
- may play a role in preventing and treating depression
- contribute to the normal development of the fetal brain

Minerals

Different minerals have different benefits. This means that no mineral can be termed as more beneficial or less beneficial than another. All minerals, even trace ones, are critical for the proper functioning of the body. Most of the minerals aid in body metabolism, water balance, and bone health, but they can participate in hundreds of other small ways to effectively boost health as well.

Boron: This mineral plays an essential part in bone health, brain function, anti-aging practices, sexual health, preventing cancer, treating Alzheimer's disease, and reducing muscle pain.

Calcium: This vital mineral also boosts bone health (prevents osteoporosis), relieves arthritis, improves dental heath, and relieves insomnia, menopause, premenstrual syndrome, and cramps. Furthermore, it is important in preventing or treating obesity, colon cancer, acidity, heart diseases, and high blood pressure.

Chromium: This trace mineral is important for glucose uptake in the body, and as such is particularly relevant to those suffering from diabetes. It increases glucose uptake by the cells, which stimulates fatty acid and cholesterol synthesis, and although both of those things typically seem like negative components for health, they are actually essential in small levels for a functional, healthy life.

Iron: This is a key element of hemoglobin formation, body metabolism, muscle activity, anemia, brain function, immunity, insomnia, restless leg syndrome, and the regulation of body temperature. Iron's primary role in the body is in regards to the formation of hemoglobin, which guarantees circulation of the blood and oxygenation of various organ systems. Without iron, anemia sets in, which is manifested in muscle weakness, fatigue, gastrointestinal disorders, and cognitive malfunction.

Magnesium: Magnesium can treat high blood pressure, heart attack, alcoholism, bone health, cramps, diabetes, menopause, pregnancy, and asthma. It is also very important in terms of lowering anxiety and stress, and has been closely linked to a reduction in anxiety and insomnia due to its enzymatic role in releasing hormones that calm the body and induce sleep.

Iodine: This often overlooked component of health can alleviate goitre, fibrocystic breast disease, skin conditions, and cancer, while also improving hair care, protecting pregnancy, and improving body metabolism.

Iodide: This is a secondary form of iodine, but it is very important in terms of bodily function. It is similarly involved in overall thyroid function, and without it in the body's system, goiter will develop. Iodide is vital for producing thyroxine (T4), without which the body can experience a fall in metabolic rate and an increase in cholesterol levels.

Phosphorus: This mineral is integral in reducing muscle weakness, improving bone health, boosting brain function, correcting sexual weakness, aiding in dental care, and optimizing body metabolism.

Manganese: Manganese plays an important role in the management of body metabolism, osteoporosis, reducing fatigue, reproduction, sprains, inflammation, brain function, and epilepsy.

Copper: This common mineral improves brain function, soothes arthritis, helps in skin care, eliminates throat infections, corrects hemoglobin deficiency, prevents heart diseases, and boosts immunity. It is commonly associated with the uptake of iron and the facilitation of a properly functioning circulatory system.

Potassium: Potassium can correct low blood sugar, regulate blood pressure, prevent heart diseases, increase water flow in the body, alleviate muscle disorders and cramps, boost brain function, manage diabetes, correct kidney disorders, and manage arthritis. As a vasodilator, it reduces the tension in the blood vessels and ensures the proper distribution of oxygen to vital organ systems while protecting against cardiovascular diseases. It has also been shown to boost brain function.

Selenium: Selenium might be a rare mineral, but its function is significant. It is one of the most powerful mineral antioxidants, and it actually prevents the formation of new free radicals by participating in various cellular reactions that lower the peroxide concentration in the cellular body. Reducing free radical formation is only one of selenium's functions. It also is essential for bone growth along with calcium, copper, and zinc.

Silicon: This mineral is an important player in bone health, skin care, hair care, nail health, sleep disorders, atherosclerosis, tissue development, dental care, and tuberculosis.

Sodium: This widely used mineral is a key to water balance, preventing sunstroke, improving brain function, relieving muscle cramps, and preventing premature aging.

Zinc: The final mineral on the list is very good at managing skin care, eczema, acne, healing of wounds, prostate disorders, cold, weight loss, pregnancy, reproduction, hair care, appetite loss, eye care, and night blindness. It is an essential component of more than ten important enzymatic functions of the body. Without zinc, the body will quickly lose overall function, resulting in a number of health concerns including an inability to heal wounds, store insulin, fight off disease, develop proper growth patterns, as well as defend against a variety of skin infections.

Dietary Supplements

In an ideal world, no one would need dietary supplements. Our balanced diets would provide all the vitamins, minerals, and other nutrients our bodies need. But alas, the world of American eating is far from ideal. And that, some nutrition experts and supplement advocates argue, is why we need dietary supplements. The latest federal data show that more than half of US adults use dietary supplements, mostly multivitamins. But do we really need all those pills?

The latest version of the federal Dietary Guidelines for Americans urges us to get our nutrients primarily from food:

> A fundamental premise of the Dietary Guidelines is that nutrients should come primarily from foods. Foods in nutrient-dense, mostly intact forms contain not only the essential vitamins and minerals that are often contained in nutrient supplements, but also dietary fiber and other naturally occurring substances that may have positive health effects [26].

The Following Lists Some Dietary Supplements and Their Significance:

Iron: Women who are able to become pregnant need more iron, especially heme iron, which the body absorbs more readily than nonheme iron. Heme iron is found in lean meat and poultry; nonheme iron is in white beans, lentils, spinach, enriched breads, and cereals. Foods rich in Vitamin C can aid iron absorption. Adult males need just 8 mg of iron per day; women need 18 mg, and pregnant women need 27 mg.

Folate: Women who can bear children also should eat more foods containing folate, such as beans, peas, oranges, orange juice, and dark-green leafy vegetables such as spinach, kale, and mustard greens. Because folate and folic acid (the nutrient's synthetic form) help prevent neural-tube defects in infants, women who can become pregnant should consume 400 micrograms of folic acid (from fortified foods or supplements); pregnant women should consume 600 mcg of folic acid daily.

Vitamin B12: Some people age fifty and older have trouble absorbing Vitamin B12 from food. To compensate, they should increase consumption of cereals fortified with this vitamin or take the appropriate supplements. Because B12 occurs naturally only in animal-based protein, vegetarians and vegans also should eat fortified cereals or take supplements. Most adults need 2.4 mcg per day.

Food Groups

What we eat every day determines how well our body is fueled and how efficiently it functions. Eating a clean, balanced diet with healthy choices from every group is essential to good health. You should consider eating a wide variety of grains, fruits, vegetables, protein, and dairy each and every day. Below, I've outlined the benefits of each food group.

Grains

Eating grains, especially whole grains, provides numerous vital health benefits. The fiber in whole grains helps provide a feeling of fullness without adding calories.

What can grains do?

- Reduce the risk of some chronic diseases
- Reduce blood cholesterol levels
- Lower the risk of heart disease, obesity, and type 2 diabetes
- Help with weight loss and weight management
- Prevent constipation

Protein

Meat, poultry, fish, beans and peas, eggs, nuts, and seeds supply many nutrients. These nutrients include protein, B vitamins (niacin, thiamin, riboflavin, and B6), vitamin E, iron, zinc, and magnesium.

Why protein?

- Proteins function as building blocks for bones, muscles, cartilage, skin, and blood. They are also building blocks for enzymes, hormones, and vitamins.

- B vitamins found in this food group serve a variety of functions in the body. They help release energy, play a vital role in the function of the nervous system, aid in the formation of red blood cells, and help build tissues.
- Iron is used to carry oxygen in the blood. Many teenage girls and women in their child-bearing years have iron-deficiency anemia. They should eat foods high in heme iron (meats) or eat other nonheme-iron-containing foods along with a food rich in vitamin C, which can improve absorption of nonheme iron.
- Magnesium is used in building bones and in releasing energy from muscles.
- Zinc is necessary for biochemical reactions and helps the immune system function properly.
- EPA and DHA are omega-3 fatty acids found in varying amounts in seafood. Eating eight ounces per week of seafood may help reduce the risk for heart disease.

Fruits

Fruits are great sources of many vitamins, minerals, and antioxidants that may help protect you from chronic diseases. In the long run, the health benefits of fruits guarantee you optimum health and a well-built body. Fruits also benefit your body immensely, as they are natural sources of vitamins and minerals, which are essential for the proper functioning of the body. Rich in dietary fiber, fruits also help to improve the functioning of the digestive tract. Fruits are an important part of a healthy diet for those who want to lose weight, providing ample energy and nearly every nutrient that your body needs to curb weight gain, without adding any unnecessary fats.

Moreover, fruits help you to stay away from health complications like heat stroke, high blood pressure, cancer, heart ailments, and diabetes. Fruits effectively fight skin disorders and promote healthy hair growth. It is always suggested to eat fruits in the raw form, fresh and ripe. Doing so allows you to experience their full health benefits, rather than consuming them after processing or cooking, which leaches out vitamins and minerals.

How do fruits help?

- Keep nutrient levels required by the body from being depleted
- Boost immune system—helpful for those with ongoing disease or illnesses and to prevent their occurrence
- Fruits are a "fast food"; simply pick and eat (unlike processed fast foods, which are devoid of nutrients or have a negative impact on the body)
- Keep the body at optimal function
- Are thought to promote emotional well-being among young adults
- Research suggests that eating fruits regularly correlates with other positive food choices

Vegetables

The benefits of vegetables are legendary. Tomatoes have been used as far back as 2,500 years ago by the Aztec Empire in both cuisine and medicinal purposes. Cucumbers have been part of human history for over 4,000 years; onions are thought to go back at least 5,000 years ago to their use in China, and in Greece they were used as a salve to increase strength. Vegetables have been with us for a long time, and thankfully today our awareness of the benefits of vegetables has progressed to an increased understanding of how they benefit us [28].

What are the benefits of vegetables?

- According to the CDC, "vegetables of different colors giv[e] your body a wide range of valuable nutrients, like fiber, folate, potassium, and vitamins A and C" [29].
  - Eat a variety of different-colored vegetables

- High-fiber diets decrease the risk of coronary artery disease
  - Examples of high-fiber vegetables include beans, lentils, and artichokes
- Diets with adequate folate may reduce a woman's risk of having a child with a brain or spinal cord defect
  - Examples of high-folate vegetables include black-eyed peas, cooked spinach, great northern beans, and asparagus
- Diets rich in potassium may help to maintain a healthy blood pressure
  - Examples include sweet potatoes, tomatoes, beet greens, white potatoes, white beans, lima beans, and cooked greens

Dairy

Dairy items have impressive levels of two things many of us need more of: calcium and protein. According to the CDC, the intake of dairy products is linked to improved bone health and may reduce the risk of osteoporosis. We also know that the intake of dairy products is also associated with a reduced risk of cardiovascular disease, type 2 diabetes, and lower blood pressure in adults.

Vitamin D functions in the body to maintain proper levels of calcium and phosphorous, thereby helping to build and maintain bones. Milk and soy milk fortified with vitamin D are good sources of this nutrient. Other sources include vitamin-D-fortified yogurt and vitamin-D-fortified ready-to-eat breakfast cereals.

What are the takeaways from dairy?

- Choose milk and soy milk fortified with vitamin D
- Choose yogurt and cereals fortified with vitamin D
- Dairy products are high in calcium and protein
- Their use is associated with reduced risk of cardiovascular disease, type 2 diabetes, and high blood pressure

Fats

Fats are essential to good health, and you need to consume some every day for your body processes to work efficiently. Fat is a dense energy source and a necessary nutrient for using fat-soluble vitamins (A, D, E, K). Additionally, fat in the diet helps with growth, brain and nervous system function, healthy skin, bone protection, insulation, and cushioning your organs. But not all fats are the same or provide the same health benefits.

All foods containing fats have a varying mixture of saturated, monounsaturated, and polyunsaturated fats. The Academy of Nutrition and Dietetics recommends that healthy adults should consume fats at a range of 20 to 35 percent of their total daily energy intake. They also recommend an increased consumption of n-3 polyunsaturated fatty acids and limited intake of saturated and trans fats [30]. All fats provide nine calories per gram, but depending on if they are in concentrated oil form or solid, the per-tablespoon calories change. On average, a tablespoon of oil is about 120 calories. Whether the fats you eat are in liquid form, like oil, or solid form, like margarine, they become broken down by your body into fatty acids and glycerol. Your body then takes these and forms other lipids in the body and stores the remainder in the form of a triglyceride.

Fats can be saturated or unsaturated depending on how many hydrogen atoms link to each carbon in their chemical chains. The more hydrogens attached to the chain, the more saturated the fat will be. If there are hydrogen atoms missing, the fatty acid is considered unsaturated.

Saturated Fats

Saturated fats are fatty acids that have hydrogens at all the points on their chemical chain. They are associated with triggering the liver to make more total cholesterol and more LDL cholesterol. However, recently there has been a big move to reanalyze if saturated fat is actually as bad as previously thought. Saturated fats, like palmitic acid or steric acid, seem to have different effects on LDL cholesterol circulating in your blood. Some question if enough research has been done to determine if diets low in saturated fat have any benefit or reduce your risk of heart disease. More research will be needed to understand the effect of saturated fat in the diet; however, the majority of nutrition experts, including the Academy of Nutrition and Dietetics, still recommends keeping saturated fat to a minimum in the diet.

Sources of saturated fat

- Meats
- Butter
- Whole milk
- Poultry
- Coconut oil
- Palm oil

Unsaturated Fats

Unsaturated fats fall into two categories: monounsaturated and polyunsaturated. Monounsaturated and polyunsaturated fats are considered to be more health beneficial than saturated fats or trans fats.

Monounsaturated fatty acids (MUFAs) are fatty acids that are missing one hydrogen pair on their chain. They are associated with lowering LDL cholesterol, total cholesterol, and at the same time increasing the production of the "good" cholesterol, HDL cholesterol. These fats are usually liquid at room temperature.

Good sources

- Sunflower oil
- Canola oil
- Olive oil
- Peanut oil
- Hazelnuts
- Macadamia nuts
- Avocados

Polyunsaturated fatty acids (PUFAs) are missing two or more hydrogen pairs on their fatty acid chains. They trigger lower blood/serum cholesterol as well as lower LDL production. However, they have also been shown to lower HDL production. Recall that generally speaking, LDL is considered bad cholesterol, while HDL is considered good. These fats are usually liquid at room temperature.

Good sources

- Flaxseed oil
- Corn oil
- Sesame oil
- Sunflower seeds and sunflower oil
- Fatty fish, i.e., salmon
- Walnuts

Some specific polyunsaturated fatty acids of a different structure with important health benefits include omega-3 fatty acids and omega-6 fatty acids.

Omega-3s are found in meat sources. In nonmeat sources, our bodies process alpha-linolenic acid into usable omega-3s. These fats are considered especially health beneficial because they are linked with improving immunity, rheumatoid arthritis, vision, brain function, and heart health. Omega-3s have been shown to lower both triglyceride levels in the body and total cholesterol levels. It is recommended that you consume foods rich in omega-3s frequently.

Good sources

- Seafood, i.e., high-fat mackerel, albacore tuna, sardines, salmon, lake trout
- Flaxseed oil
- Walnuts
- Soybean oil
- Canola oil

Omega-6 fatty acids found in vegetable oils are also PUFAs. They are also associated with reducing cardiovascular disease risk by lowering LDL cholesterol levels. However, they may also lower HDL levels.

Good sources

- Most vegetable oils
- Sunflower seeds
- Pine nuts

Trans Fats

Trans fats are created when food manufacturers extend the shelf life of foods with fats in them by adding hydrogen to their chemical makeup. Adding hydrogen makes the fats in the food firmer and more saturated, thereby delaying rancidity and extending freshness. Sadly, trans fats are linked to increasing total cholesterol and LDL cholesterol, as well as lowering HDL cholesterol. This cholesterol profile (high LDL and low HDL) is a deadly combination.

You will find small amounts of trans fats naturally occurring in beef, pork, butter, and milk. However, these trans fats have different effects from the man-made trans fats and are not associated with having the same effects on cholesterol levels.

How to Read Food Labels

Most of the prepacked edibles have food labels on them. These labels are meant for providing the complete information of the basic ingredients. A label provides information regarding the amount of energy (in kilojoules and kilocalories) of a food item, usually expressed as calories. The label also provides information regarding fats (e.g., saturated, mono-, or polyunsaturated), carbohydrates (e.g., sugars), minerals, and proteins.

How a Food Label Is Structured

Below is an example of the typical food label. The information is provided per 100g by default or per portion of that food. The label is broken down for you by its components, a few of which are placed in bold type because of their significance. These important components include caloric value, fats, saturated fats, salts, and sugars. Extra attention (bolding) is done to stress these specific components because excess of these may be harmful for some people. If you want a balanced diet, you ought to know exactly what you are eating.

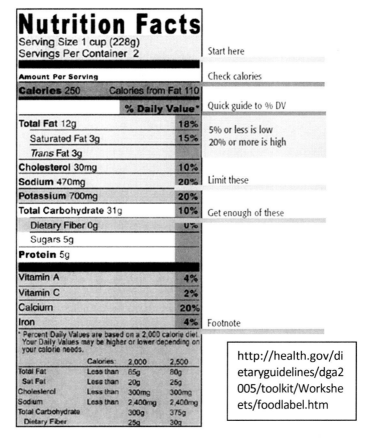

How to Read Food Labels

The image above shows a typical food label. It has different parts which are labeled and explained next page.

1. General Information

Label reading should be started with the general information about the edible given on the top of the label. Note that the serving size and the servings per container in the above example are 2/3 of a cup, which equals 55g, and 8 servings respectively.

2. Caloric Value

Check the total number of calories present. It is important to adjust your caloric intake according to your lifestyle and physical activities. You'll recall that unless we remain physically active, as we age our caloric requirement is significantly less. If you are in this latter category, be sure to lower your total daily caloric intake to reflect your comparatively lower metabolism.

3. Limit the Intake of These Nutrients

These nutritional elements are harmful when taken in higher concentration. You have to limit the intake of fats, carbohydrates, and sodium.

4. These Nutrients Are Beneficial

These nutrients, e.g., proteins, calcium, dietary fibers, iron, vitamins, etc., are beneficial for the body. Foods rich in these are considered healthier than those that are deficient in them. Generally speaking, foods that have high amounts of nutrients in this category are a better choice than those foods with high amounts of elements in category 3.

5. Percent Daily Value

This portion of the label guides you in understanding what proportion the different constituents are of your daily recommended amount of that component. For example, in the label above you will note that there are 8gm of total fat per serving, which is 12 percent of your daily value of total fat. This means that for a 2,000 calorie diet, you should eat no more than 65 grams of total fat. To check this yourself, you may use the following word problem:

8gm is what percent of 65g?

$8 = (x \text{ percent}) \times 65$

$x = 12 \text{ percent}$

In Conclusion: A Word to Readers

My hope is that you will find the first half of this chapter a helpful place to begin your learning about nutrition. There is a great deal to learn in this area; it is, after all, an entire field of study upon which careers are built. Please take the time to revisit the material that I've included as a reference. With regards to further education, feel free to use this material as a springboard for searching for other existing work on these subjects. Take, for example, the sources for credible nutrition information that I've cited as a starting point. Once you've located them on the internet, spend some time searching their websites for topics that I've discussed in this chapter. You will find a great deal of information, some of which may be specific to areas of concern that you will find important and applicable to your situation. As always, seek clarification from your physician or other trusted health professional, while at the same time trusting and empowering yourself with real, actionable intelligence.

Run for Your Life—Exercise Basics

If you're waiting for a magic pill that will melt the fat away, keep the weight off, and keep your body at full health, stop now. You've wasted enough time. Along with the proper hydration and nutrition, God has designed your body to naturally burn fat and build muscle as you exercise it. Your body is a gift from God that keeps on giving if you treat it right. It is possible to achieve a strong, healthy, beautifully shaped body that is full of energy and vitality for a lifetime.

But if you're among the 50 percent of Americans who live a totally sedentary lifestyle, you're not giving your body a chance to function in the healthy way in which God designed it. Despite repeated warnings from the surgeon general and the National Center for Chronic Disease Prevention, millions of Americans are suffering from illnesses that can be prevented or improved through regular exercise. Far too many of us continue to pay the price for consuming more calories than we burn and for abusing our body through lack of care.

There's a simple reason why exercise is such a powerful key to weight loss. Exercise burns calories, and when calories are burned, the body compensates for the extra energy used. Compensation occurs as the mitochondria, or power plants, inside your body cells divide, burning twice as many calories. Nothing else will do that.

According to the National Institutes of Health, regular exercise and physical activity are important to the physical and mental health of almost everyone, including older adults [32]. Being physically active can help you continue to do the things you enjoy and stay independent as you age. Regular physical activity over long periods of time can produce numerous long-term health benefits. That is why health experts say that older adults should be active every day to maintain their health.

In addition, regular exercise and physical activity can reduce the risk of developing some diseases and disabilities that develop as people age. In some cases, exercise is an effective treatment for many chronic conditions. For example, studies show that people with arthritis, heart disease, or diabetes benefit from regular exercise. Exercise also helps those with high blood pressure, balance problems, or anyone having difficulty walking.

The Most Useful Forms of Activity and Exercise

Experts tell us that the following activities represent the main types of exercise you want to get at any age:

- **Aerobic**: Good for your heart and lungs. Increases your breathing and heart rate. Examples include brisk walking, jogging, swimming, biking, tennis, and dancing.
- **Flexibility and Balance**: Helps prevent falls. Examples include walking up and down stairs, standing on one foot, yoga, and tai chi.
- **Strength Training**: Promotes muscle and bone health. Examples include lifting weights and performing daily activities, such as carrying a full laundry basket, carrying your smaller grandchildren, or lifting things in the garden.

Specific Benefits to Your Health and Well-Being

A report in the Journal of the American Medical Associaton in 2015 showed that mature adults who maintain or begin any type of physical activity appear to live longer and have a lower risk of disability [33]. Likewise, experts from the National Institute on Aging (NIA) [32] indicate that in addition to helping your fitness, stamina, balance, and muscle and bone strength, physical activity and exercise can also:

- Improve your mood and help with feelings of depression or anxiety
- Maintain your thinking skills
- Make it easier to do the things you want to do
- Help prevent or treat diseases such as diabetes, heart disease, high blood pressure, breast and colon cancer, and osteoporosis

For all of these reasons, many people of retirement age are seeking a lifestyle that offers plentiful opportunities to stay active, engaged, and healthy.

Aerobic and Endurance Exercise

Aerobic exercise is key for your head, just as it is for your heart. You may not agree at first; indeed, the first steps are the hardest, and in the beginning, exercise will be more work than fun. But as you get into shape, you'll begin to tolerate exercise, then enjoy it, and finally depend on it.

Regular aerobic exercise will bring remarkable changes to your body, your metabolism, your heart, and your spirits. It has a unique capacity to exhilarate and relax, to provide stimulation and calm, to counter depression and dissipate stress. It's a common experience among endurance athletes and has been verified in clinical trials that have successfully used exercise to treat anxiety disorders and clinical depression [36]. If athletes and patients can derive psychological benefits from exercise, so can you.

How can exercise contend with problems as difficult as anxiety and depression? There are several explanations, some chemical and others behavioral.

The mental benefits of aerobic exercise have a neurochemical basis. Exercise reduces levels of the body's stress hormones, such as adrenaline and cortisol. It also stimulates the production of endorphins, chemicals in the brain that are the body's natural painkillers and mood elevators. Endorphins are responsible for the "runner's high" and for the feelings of relaxation and optimism that accompany many hard workouts—or, at least, the hot shower after your exercise is over.

Behavioral factors also contribute to the emotional benefits of exercise. As your waistline shrinks and your strength and stamina increase, your self-image will improve. You'll earn a sense of mastery and control, of pride and self-confidence. Your renewed vigor and energy will help you succeed in many tasks, and the discipline of regular exercise will help you achieve other important lifestyle goals.

Exercise and sports also provide opportunities to get away from it all and to either enjoy some solitude or to make friends and build networks. To paraphrase St. Thomas Aquinas, all men need leisure. Exercise is play and recreation; when your body is busy, your mind will be distracted from the worries of daily life and will be free to think creatively.

Almost any type of exercise will help. Many people find that using large muscle groups in a rhythmic, repetitive fashion works best; call it "muscular meditation," and you'll begin to understand how it works. Walking and jogging are prime examples. Even a simple twenty-minute stroll can clear the mind and reduce stress. Other people prefer vigorous workouts that burn stress along with calories. That's one reason ellipticals are so popular. Furthermore, those same stretching exercises that help relax your muscles after a hard workout will help relax your mind as well.

Autoregulation Exercises

Stress comes in many forms and produces many symptoms. Mental symptoms range from worry and irritability to restlessness and insomnia, anger and hostility, or sensations of dread, foreboding, and even panic. Mental stress can also produce physical symptoms: tense muscles resulting in fidgetiness, taut facial expressions, headaches, or neck and back pain. Stress also causes a dry mouth, even producing unquenchable thirst, or perhaps the sensation of a lump in the throat that makes swallowing difficult. Clenched jaw muscles can produce jaw pain and headaches. The skin can become pale, sweaty, and clammy. Intestinal symptoms during stress range from "butterflies" to heartburn, cramps, or diarrhea. Frequent urination may also be a bother. A pounding pulse is common, as is chest tightness. Rapid breathing may occur, accompanied by sighing or repetitive coughing. In extreme cases, hyperventilation can lead to tingling of the face and fingers, or muscle cramps, lightheadedness, and even fainting.

The physical symptoms of stress are themselves distressing. In fact, the body's response to stress can feel so bad that it produces additional mental stress. During the stress response, then, mind and body can amplify each other's distress signals, creating a vicious cycle of tension and anxiety.

Because the root cause of stress is emotional, it is best controlled by gaining insight, reducing life problems that trigger stress, and modifying behavior. However, stress control can and should also involve the body. Aerobic exercise is one great approach to stress control; physical fitness will help promote mental fitness. But there is also another approach: you can learn to use your mind to relax your body. The relaxed body will, in turn, send signals of calm and control that help reduce mental tension.

Autoregulation exercises are a group of techniques designed to replace the spiral of stress with a cycle of repose. Several approaches are available.

Breathing Exercises

Even without formal meditation and controlled breathing, the gentle muscle stretching of yoga can reduce stress. "Full service" yoga is even better. But if that's not your thing, simple breathing exercises can help by themselves. Rapid, shallow, erratic breathing is a common response to stress. Slow, deep, regular breathing is a sign of relaxation. You can learn to control your respirations so they mimic relaxation; the effect, in fact, will be relaxing.

Here's how deep breathing exercises work:

1. Breathe in slowly and deeply, pushing your stomach out so that your diaphragm is put to maximal use.
2. Hold your breath briefly.
3. Exhale slowly, thinking "relax."
4. Repeat the entire sequence five to ten times, concentrating on breathing deeply and slowly.

Deep breathing is easy to learn. You can do it at any time, in any place. You can use deep breathing to help dissipate stress as it occurs. Practice the routine in advance, then use it when you need it most. If you find this practice helpful, consider repeating the exercise four to six times a day—even on good days.

Mental exercises, too

Bodily exercise can help relax the mind and mental maneuvers can, too. Most often, that means talking out problems with a supportive listener, who can be a friend, a chaplain, or a trained counselor or psychotherapist. But you can also do it yourself, harnessing the power of your own mind to reduce stress. Simply writing down your thoughts and feelings can be very beneficial, and formal meditation exercises have helped many people reduce stress and gain perspective.

Meditation is a prime example of the unity of mind and body. Mental stress can speed up the heart and raise blood pressure; meditation can actually reverse the physiological signs of stress. Scientific studies of Indian yoga masters demonstrate that meditation can, in fact, slow the heart rate, lower blood pressure, reduce the breathing rate, diminish the body's oxygen consumption, reduce blood adrenaline levels, and change skin temperature.

Although meditation is an ancient Eastern religious technique, you don't have to become a pilgrim or convert to put it to work for you. Here's an outline of what is termed as the relaxation response:

1. Select a time and place that will be free of distractions and interruption. A semidarkened room is often best; it should be quiet and private. If possible, wait two hours after you eat before you meditate and empty your bladder before you get started.
2. Get comfortable. Find a body position that will allow your body to relax so that physical signals of discomfort will not intrude on your mental processes. Breathe slowly and deeply, allowing your mind to become aware of your rhythmic respirations.
3. Achieve a relaxed, passive mental attitude. Close your eyes to block out visual stimuli. Try to let your mind go blank, blocking out thoughts and worries.
4. Concentrate on a mental device. Most people use a mantra, a simple word or syllable that is repeated over and over again in a rhythmic, chant-like fashion. You can repeat your mantra silently or say it aloud. It's the act of repetition that counts, not the content of the phrase; even the word "one" will do nicely. Some meditators prefer to stare at a fixed object instead of repeating a mantra. In either case, the goal is to focus your attention on a neutral object, thus blocking out ordinary thoughts and sensations.

Meditation is the most demanding of the autoregulation techniques, but it's also the most beneficial and rewarding. Once you've mastered meditation, you'll probably look forward to devoting twenty minutes to it once or twice a day.

Progressive Muscular Relaxation

Stressed muscles are tight, tense muscles. By learning to relax your muscles, you will be able to use your body to dissipate stress. This method, muscle relaxation, takes a bit longer to learn than deep breathing. It also takes more time. But even if this form of relaxation takes a little effort, it can be a useful part of your stress control program. Here's how it works:

Progressive muscle relaxation is best performed in a quiet, secluded place. You should be comfortably seated or stretched out on a firm mattress or mat. Until you learn the routine, have a friend recite the directions or listen to them on a tape, which you can prerecord yourself.

Progressive muscle relaxation focuses sequentially on the major muscle groups. Tighten each muscle and maintain the contraction twenty seconds before slowly releasing it. As the muscle relaxes, concentrate on the release of tension and the sensation of relaxation. Start with your facial muscles, then work down the body.

Exercise, Health, and Stress

Few things are more stressful than illness. Many forms of exercise reduce stress directly, and by preventing bodily illness, exercise has extra benefits for the mind. Regular physical activity will lower your blood pressure, improve your cholesterol, and reduce your blood sugar. Exercise cuts the risk of heart attack, stroke, diabetes, colon and breast cancers, osteoporosis and fractures, obesity, depression, and even dementia (memory loss). Exercise also slows the aging process, increases energy, and prolongs life.

Except during illness, you should exercise nearly every day. That doesn't necessarily mean hitting the gym or training for a marathon. But it does mean thirty to forty minutes of moderate exercise, such as walking, or fifteen to twenty minutes of vigorous exercise. More is even better, but the first steps provide the most benefit. Aim to walk at least two miles a day, or do the equivalent amount of another activity. You can do it all at once or in ten- to fifteen-minute chunks if that fits your schedule better. Add a little strength training and stretching two to three times a week, and you'll have an excellent, balanced program for health and stress reduction. And if you need more help with stress, consider autoregulation exercises involving deep breathing or muscular relaxation. Remember, too, that mental exercises are the time-honored ways to cut stress.

How Much Exercise Is Needed for Fitness?

In 2001, ACSM recommended that overweight and obese adults get at least 150 minutes of moderate-intensity exercise per week to improve their health. Two hundred to three hundred minutes per week was recommended for long-term weight loss [31]. But will this amount of exercise really help you lose weight and keep it off?

New research shows that between 150 and 250 minutes per week of moderate intensity physical activity is effective in preventing weight gain greater than 3 percent in most adults, but will provide "only modest" weight loss [37]. So ACSM has published new physical activity recommendations in the journal *Medicine & Science in Sports & Exercise*. Their recommendations are that overweight and obese individuals are more likely to lose weight and keep it off if they exercise for least 250 minutes per week. Exercising for more than 250 minutes per week has resulted in "significant" weight loss for these individuals [38].

Exercise for Different Age Groups

Ages 10–20

A wide range of activities is preferable, and building up as much bone mineral density as possible is vital. Hopping, running, skipping, jumping off things, and rapid twisting are all important.

Weight training was previously thought to be detrimental to the physical development of adolescents, but there has recently been a substantial shift in thinking, as exercising with weights is known to increase bone density.

Ages 20–30

It is still important to develop bone mineral density at this age, so the ideal activities are weight bearing and dynamic, such as running, dancing, football, or martial arts. It is also good to do some posture work, such as Pilates, yoga, Alexander technique, or balancing exercises on a FitBall (or Swiss ball). Anything involving balance is good, and it doesn't have to be a formal, organised activity; dance, for example, is great.

Ages 30–40

It is possible to play top-class sports until the midthirties. It is important to do short, intense bursts of activity at this age, rather than thinking that fitness is all about building endurance. Whatever cardiovascular activity you do, be it indoor rowing, running, swimming, or triathlon, make sure you also do strength training. You can lose loads of weight doing endurance work, but weight training develops the whole body.

Ages 40–50

The fifth decade is when our bodies express, ever more loudly, what they have been put through. Joint wear and tear is commonplace, with signs of osteoarthritis often coming to light. Given that lung function declines with age, it is important to maintain cardiovascular fitness. If your knees are painful, then swim, cycle, or use an indoor rower. Whatever the state of your joints, this is a good time to undergo gait analysis, which involves running on a treadmill while a sports-injury specialist, aided by a bundle of computer software, assesses postural abnormalities.

Ages 50–60

Investment for later life is the mantra as we approach retirement age. Nerve conduction and reflexes slow down as we age. A classic cause of disability in elderly people is falling due to loss of balance. Pilates, Alexander technique, and core stability exercises can work wonders in training the neural system. Strength training is a must, too. Use lighter weights or rubber resistance bands instead. Aim for twenty to thirty repeats.

Ages 60–70

Between the ages of thirty and seventy, the average person loses 25 percent of their muscle mass [39]. In this decade alone, they lose 15 percent of their strength. Relatively speaking, though, endurance increases, hence the number of veteran runners in marathons. While it could be argued that it would make sense to go in for plodding, ultradistance challenges to boost fitness levels, working on weaknesses, i.e., strength, should take priority.

Ages 70–80

Our metabolism slows down as we become older and we require a lower caloric intake. This should be considered when we exercise—otherwise, that post-workout hunger could result in excess calories and increased body fat.

Types of Exercises

The National Institutes of Health (NIH) recommends four types of exercises for optimum health and well-being: strength, balance, stretching, and endurance.

Strength

Strength exercises retain and build muscles and increase metabolism. With strength exercises, we can help keep our weight down and blood-sugar in check. A reduced schedule, which is common in older age or just with time off, can sometimes lead to less activity. The key to staying strong when life slows down is to keep doing strength exercises. Exercise can build muscles and keep older people independent. For best results, we should start slow. Some examples of good strength exercises are:

- Knee flexions
- Chair stands
- Arm raises
- Bicep curls
- Tricep extensions

Stretching

With increasing age, our muscles become shorter and lose their elasticity, along with decreased range of motion in the shoulders, spine, and hips. Stretching exercises can give more freedom of movement and help keep them flexible. For aged people, the National Institute on Aging recommends regularly stretching the neck, shoulders, upper arms, upper body, chest, back, ankles, legs, hips, and calves. They can start with a few stretching exercises each day, building up to all the areas.

Balance

Balance exercises build leg muscles and keep us in practice for movements that use muscles that, while we may not use them all the time, must still be kept active. These muscles are critical in helping to prevent falls, especially in old age. According to the NIH, US hospitals have over 300,000 admissions for broken hips each year, many of them seniors, and falling is often the cause of those fractures [39]. Balance exercises will help loved ones avoid many more serious problems that are often started with an injury. Balance exercises include:

- Chair-supported, single-leg balancing
- Eye tracking
- Clock reach
- Staggered stance
- Chair-supported single leg with arm
- Balancing wand
- Knee marching
- Body circles
- Heel to toe
- Grapevine
- Stepping exercises
- Dynamic walking

Endurance

Endurance exercises are any activity—walking, jogging, swimming, biking, even raking leaves or mopping floors—that increases heart rate and elevates breathing for an extended period of time. We should work toward getting at least thirty minutes of activity that makes us breathe hard on most or all days of the week.

How to Start Exercising

Our lifestyles have changed dramatically. With ever-increasing advances in technology, we have become less physically active. The most prevalent diseases we suffer from today, i.e., heart disease, stroke, and cancer, are related to our lifestyles, of which adequate physical activity should be a major part. It is as essential as sleep and nourishment. Although many of us know that exercising will reduce the risk of disease and illness, the thought of exercise can still be overwhelming. Myths that contribute to an inactive lifestyle are that exercise has to be difficult, it has to hurt, and you have to do lots of it for it to be beneficial. These are all false. Exercise is about enjoying a physically active lifestyle (e.g., walking or cycling to the shops rather than driving) that includes increasing your heart rate (such as brisk walking) a few times a week.

If you have heart disease, high blood pressure, back problems, arthritis, joint pain, diabetes, are recovering from an illness or are pregnant, check with your doctor before starting any exercise regimen.

Some of the benefits of exercise are:

- Reduced risk of heart disease
- Reduced risk of high blood pressure
- Decreased resting heart rate (so your heart doesn't have to work as hard)
- Increased bone density
- Reduced risk of osteoporosis
- Improved strength and stamina
- Increased coordination and balance (especially important for older adults)
- Improved flexibility
- Improved respiration
- Improved circulation
- Help with preventing constipation
- Help with weight control
- Improved sense of well-being and reduced stress

Four Critical Aspects of Exercise

1. Cardiovascular fitness

This refers to the fitness level of your heart, lungs, veins, and arteries, which are responsible for processing and transporting oxygen to your muscles. As your fitness improves, your heart will become more efficient, being able to pump more blood with fewer contractions. This is what is meant by a reduced or slower resting heart rate. A slow resting heart rate means your heart is working with ease and efficiency, while a high resting heart rate means that your heart is having to work hard.

A couple of points to increase your understanding: your resting heart rate is the number of heartbeats per minute from the time you first wake up and before you get up to stand; also, exercises which use oxygen (i.e., aerobic exercises) are those that improve cardiovascular fitness. In other words, being cardiovascularly fit means that you have pursued enough of the types of exercise that elevate your heart rate to the point of needing to breathe hard that when you are at rest, your heart rate is low. Some serious athletes who achieved superior cardiovascular fitness have resting heart rates as low as forty beats per minute.

2. Muscular strength and 3. Endurance

If you do not use your muscles, they will shrink. Muscular strength is necessary to perform fundamental movements of everyday life: lifting your children, carrying your shopping, even standing. Endurance (stamina) is necessary to continue to walk or carry your shopping without becoming tired. Both are essential in order to maintain mobility and functionality, particularly in older age. Without them, we cannot live an independent life. Furthermore, muscular tissue uses more calories than inactive tissue, which is good news for those trying to control their weight. Resistance exercises improve muscular strength and endurance.

4. Flexibility

Flexibility is critical, yet often overlooked. Flexibility is the range of movement at a joint (where two or more bones meet). Without flexibility, we suffer from increased stiffness, poor posture, and muscular tension, particularly in older age. If you've ever experienced great stiffness when trying to turn around from a seated position to parallel park, you know exactly what I mean. Not only does increased flexibility help with simple daily tasks, it also helps to reduce the possibility of injury and the risk of lower back pain. Exercises to improve flexibility include stretching and yoga.

How to Exercise

Becoming physically active is about incorporating exercise into our daily routine (discussed later) and increasing cardiovascular fitness, strength, endurance, and flexibility. There are some basic principles of exercise which will ensure that you gain the maximum benefit from your exercise and that you exercise safely. These principles concern how often you should exercise, for how long, and how difficult the exercise should be. Also to consider is the fact that exercise should include a warm-up, a cooldown, and a thorough stretching of the muscles that you are going to use. Having this basic understanding about exercise will make it more enjoyable and help keep you motivated.

Warming Up and Cooling Down

Depending on your exercise, your warm-up and cooldown could be the same activity performed at a less intense level. For example, if you planned a walk, walk at a slower pace for your warm-up and cooldown.

Warming up:
- Increases the blood flow to the muscles
- Decreases the chances of injuries to the muscles or joints
- Should be for five to ten minutes at a very low intensity

Cooling down:
- Prevents blood pooling in your extremities, e.g., your legs
- Should be about five minutes, gradually reducing intensity level

Stretching

You should stretch your muscles after your warm-up and cooldown. Stretching is very important, as it reduces risk of injury and stiffness, makes your muscles more able to perform the exercise you're doing, and improves flexibility. A common mistake is to stretch muscles before they are warm. You must warm up first, then stretch your muscles. Stretching cold muscles could injure them. It's also a good idea to specifically stretch the muscles you are going to use in your exercise.

Breathe in and slowly and gently elongate the muscle you are stretching until you feel tension. Breathe out. If the tension is uncomfortable, find a tension that is comfortable, but aim to feel the stretch. Maintain slow, deep breaths. Hold for ten to thirty seconds, then slowly and gently come out of the stretch. Never bounce at any stage, and stop immediately if you feel pain.

When you stretch properly, the longer you hold the stretch, the less you will feel it. If you do begin to feel your muscle tighten, relax it. It is also a good idea to borrow a video demonstrating which muscles to stretch and the correct way to perform the stretches. It won't take you long to learn what to do.

How Often to Exercise

It is currently recommended that we be physically active every day, exercising aerobically three to five times a week (e.g., brisk walking, cycling, swimming). However, begin with exercising aerobically three times a week. If you have led a sedentary lifestyle until now, leave a day or two in between your exercise days so that your body can recover and equilibrate to new levels of activity. Remember, the body is always trying to achieve homeostasis (balance).

How Long to Exercise

The most widely accepted minimum length of time you should spend exercising is twenty minutes (which does not include the warm-up and cooldown). The maximum is one hour, depending on the exercise you choose. If you are a beginner, try starting with ten minutes. I'm hoping that you see the pattern here; the idea is to start slowly and gradually increase your activity time. Don't worry if all you can do is ten minutes, because that "all" is the start of a path that leads to a more productive and healthy life.

How Difficult Should the Exercise Be?

The difficulty, or intensity level, of your exercise is another essential factor to improving fitness. You may choose to walk for thirty minutes a day (sounds excellent), but you won't improve your cardiovascular fitness by taking a gentle stroll. Beginners should exercise at low intensities, and it is important that you increase the length of time you exercise before you increase the intensity. For example, if you begin walking, aim to increase the number of minutes you walk before you increase the intensity (by either increasing your speed or walking uphill).

The key to achieving the maximum benefit from your exercise, and to making sure that you exercise safely, is to measure the intensity level of your exercise. This is by no means as daunting or as difficult as it sounds. There are a number of ways to measure how hard you are exercising, ranging from a very simple subjective test (e.g., ensuring that you can still talk while you exercise) to taking your pulse, either manually or with a heart rate monitor. You can choose whichever method suits you best.

1. The talk test

The talk test method is a subjective measure to determine how hard you are exercising. If you are able to talk during your exercise without too much effort, you are within a safe level of exercise.

2. Rating perceived exertion

Another subjective measure is to rate how you feel on a scale from zero to twenty. You should be exercising between twelve (somewhat hard) to sixteen (hard). This is the method that people should use who do not have a typical heart rate response to exercise (e.g., those on beta-blocking medications, some cardiac and diabetic patients). Although this method is by no means precise, it is a way that you can self-monitor your exertion level, helping you to know when enough is enough or when to push a little more.

3. Measuring your heart rate

You can measure your heart rate manually by taking your pulse or with a heart rate monitor. Measuring your heart rate ensures that you exercise at the level that is ideal for you. If you exercise at levels that are too low, you won't improve your fitness and may become frustrated by your lack of progress. Measuring your heart rate also makes sure that you don't push yourself too hard or overexert yourself. Furthermore, you will be able to measure your progress, which is motivating, and as your fitness improves you will be able to adjust your heart rate to match your fitness, thus maintaining an optimum level of exercise.

4. Taking your pulse

Use your index and middle fingers on one hand and find the pulse on the other hand on the underside and thumb side of your wrist, just above your wrist bone. Press down lightly. If you prefer you can take your pulse from the artery to the right or left near your adam's apple. When you have found your pulse, count the number of beats, counting the first beat as zero, for either six seconds (then multiply this number by ten) or for ten seconds (then multiply this number by six) to get the number of times your heart is beating per minute. Bear in mind that although counting for six seconds is easier, the longer you count for, the more accurate your results will be. You should check your pulse about five minutes into your exercise and again five minutes before you stop. You may have to stop exercising to do this, so take it immediately, as your pulse rate will slow down rapidly.

5. Using a heart rate monitor

All you need is a basic monitor which consists of a sensor strap, which fits around your torso next to your skin, and a wrist monitor. The two communicate, and your heart rate is continuously displayed on the wrist monitor. This type of monitoring is extremely easy to use.

Although there is no initial financial cost with measuring your heart rate manually, feeling and counting your pulse can be tricky (especially during exercise) and it is less accurate than using a heart rate monitor. A heart rate monitor, however, is accurate, and your heart rate is displayed continuously, allowing you to always exercise at the absolute optimum level. The immediate feedback is also fun and motivational.

Calculating Your Intensity Level

You can easily calculate the level at which you should be exercising. Your maximum heart rate (i.e., the fastest your heart can beat) is used as the reference point for determining your intensity level. You can estimate your maximum heart rate by subtracting your age from 220. For example, if you are forty years old, 220 − 40 = 180, your maximum heart rate is 180 beats per minute (bpm). Aerobic exercise should be at levels that are between 60 percent and 85 percent of your maximum heart rate. Between this range are zones. You can match your current level of fitness and your exercise goals with the appropriate zone. This way, you achieve exactly what you want from your exercise. To achieve a wide range of benefits, you could aim to exercise at several intensities.

You can calculate your zones simply by multiplying your maximum heart rate by each percent of your zone. A good place to calculate your zone of fitness can be found at http://www.runningforfitness.org/calc/heart-rate-calculators/hrzone.

Measuring your heart rate is not a completely reliable method by itself to ensure that you don't push yourself too hard. There may be days when you find it more difficult to achieve your desired heart rate because you are tired, you have a cold, or you are feeling a bit low, for example. Rather than push yourself, take into account how you are feeling before and during your exercise session.

The Successful Combination

You have to apply the frequency, the length of time, and the intensity level of your exercise together to achieve the results you are working toward. Understanding these three things (frequency, time, and intensity) is the key to successful exercise and achieving your fitness goals. For example, if you exercise for twenty minutes at an appropriate intensity level, but only once or twice a week, you won't improve your fitness. The recommendation is twenty to sixty minutes, three to five times a week at 60 to 85 percent of your maximum heart rate.

To improve fitness, you have to work your body harder than it is used to. If you haven't done any exercise for a while, it won't take much to do this. As you become more fit, you will need to increase the frequency, intensity, and/or time of your exercise to continue to improve your fitness.

The Right Combination for You

You may prefer to exercise more often—for example, six days a week at a lower intensity—or you may prefer to exercise three to four times a week at a higher intensity. A word of caution: be careful not to overexercise, either by overexerting yourself during your exercise or exercising too often for too long at a level that is difficult for you. You can monitor the former either subjectively and/or by measuring your heart rate. The latter may make you feel tired rather than energised, so adjust your exercise pattern either by taking days out from exercise or reducing the intensity level and the amount of time you exercise. Fatigue, insomnia, and irritability are signs of exercising too much, so if you are feeling these, take a break for a day or two.

There are three other aspects of exercise: strength, endurance, and flexibility. As well as improving cardiovascular fitness, aerobic exercise can also improve strength/endurance (e.g., walking, swimming) and flexibility (by stretching after the warm-up/cooldown). Exercise classes (e.g., keep fit/aerobics) also usually combine all four aspects, so this is a great way to get all of your exercise needs met in one sitting.

There are other options to improve strength, e.g., going to a gym or joining a Pilates class. To improve flexibility, stretches can be incorporated into everyday life (e.g., when you get undressed at night or in the shower). Yoga also improves flexibility and helps with relaxation and circulation, and certain styles of yoga can also improve strength and endurance. There are so many ways to make exercise a part of your daily life. Be creative and have fun with it. Within limits, you will certainly get out what you put in. This is a reality in the fitness world.

How to Start

One of the main reasons for not exercising is not knowing where to start. Here are some tips on how to start exercising.

Each exercise session should follow this pattern: warm-up, stretch, aerobic exercise, cooldown, and stretch. Begin exercising for a short time (e.g., ten minutes) on nonconsecutive days (e.g., three days a week) with a small amount of effort.

Gradually increase the frequency, time, and/or intensity of your exercise. Increase the length of time you exercise before you increase the intensity; increase your exercise time by five- to ten-minute increments.

Choose Your Exercise

Remove as many hurdles to exercising as possible, so choose an exercise that (1) you enjoy, (2) is convenient, (3) is affordable, and (4) you can assimilate into your lifestyle. Don't be tempted to take up an exercise that you think will be "good for you" rather than one that you think is fun; it is likely to become a chore and you won't stick to it. If time is a constraint, try to choose one that is convenient, e.g., walking, jogging, cycling, or swimming. You can divide these into two sets: one before and one after work. If you have children, try taking up an activity that you can enjoy as a family, e.g., cycling.

You may not know which activity (or activities) will suit you, so take the time to try a few. You may find that you prefer to vary your activities because you either find just one form of exercise boring or that different activities on different days fits in with your lifestyle better (e.g., an aerobic class or swimming during lunch breaks/after work, walking with a friend on the weekend). If you have chosen an outdoor activity, find an indoor activity for bad weather days.

A common myth is that walking is too easy to be beneficial. Walking is an ideal form of exercise, particularly for beginners, which can make you fit as long as you walk at an appropriate level of difficulty and for enough time. Swimming is another ideal exercise. It is a gentle aerobic activity that is ideal for those who are recovering from an injury, have joint problems, or are overweight or pregnant. If you measure your heart rate, it won't get as high as with other aerobic activities, but if you swim at a level that you find somewhat hard to handle, you will still be exercising aerobically.

Choose Your Time

Decide how often you are going to exercise a week. Choose the most convenient days and times of day, and set aside those times as you would for other essential commitments.

Start Slowly

Start with small amounts of time and little effort and increase gradually. Don't try to do too much too soon, as you may feel unwell and lose motivation to continue. A key to successful exercising is to start slowly, particularly if you have led a sedentary lifestyle. You will finish your exercise with a sense of achievement, you will feel better, and you will give yourself the motivation to continue. It is also essential to start slowly to prevent injury.

Increase Gradually

With increasing levels of fitness, you will need to alter your exercise (frequency, time, and/or intensity) to make sure you are still working your body more than it is used to. It is important to increase your exercise gradually. If you make your exercise too difficult or try to increase your difficulty level too soon before you are ready, you might feel ill, begin to dislike exercising, and lose motivation to continue.

Invest in Good Equipment

If you choose to walk, it is very important to invest in a good pair of walking shoes/sneakers which offer support for your spine, hips, knees, ankles, and feet. You will also enjoy walking more with a comfortable, supportive pair of shoes. Incorporating walking into your daily activities is an excellent way to lead a more active lifestyle—by the way, for this you don't necessarily need walking shoes, but if you are going to walk for a long period of time and with effort, it is advisable to wear shoes that will support your body and make the experience more enjoyable. If you progress to jogging, it is even more essential that you invest in a pair of good running shoes.

Some other Dos and Don'ts

Don't exercise until two or three hours after a meal. It is important to drink water before, during, and after exercise to keep your body hydrated. Also, don't exercise strenuously during very hot or humid weather, as overheating (heatstroke) can occur.

Aches and Pains

During exercise, if you feel sore or ache, rest if you feel you need to. It is not unnatural to feel sore or to ache after exercise if you are just beginning or have not exercised for a while. If, however, you feel pain, stop exercising and check with your doctor.

Staying Motivated

There are going to be days when you don't feel like exercising; everybody has them. Here are some tips to help you stay motivated.

A lifestyle approach

Think of exercise as essential to your well-being like good nutrition and sleep. If something is part of your lifestyle, you do it whether you feel like it or not—like brushing your teeth. If you regard exercise as a hobby (something to be done when you feel like it), you may not exercise regularly and may lose motivation.

An ongoing process

Rather than having an all-or-nothing attitude toward exercise, think of it as an ongoing process. There may be days when you have to unavoidably miss your exercise or you may be unwell. It doesn't matter. Just continue when you can.

Set goals

Set yourself short-term goals and be realistic. In order to accomplish these goals, it is important to understand your level of fitness. The American Heart Association has developed zones of fitness based on your heart rate. The maximum heart rate is based on the formula (220 minus age) times a factor of 0.85 for women. An ideal level of fitness would be to exercise and maintain 85 to 100 percent of your target heart rate for a minimum of thirty minutes for zone 3, 65 to 85 percent for zone 2, and 50 to 65 percent for zone 1 (See source). For example, your aim may be to increase the distance you walk from ten minutes to fifteen minutes or to increase your pace so that your intensity level increases from the low end of zone 1 (50 percent of your maximum heart rate) to the high end of zone 1 (60 percent of your maximum heart rate) [35].

Reward yourself

Reward yourself when you have achieved each goal, e.g., with a small luxury or a new item of exercise clothing.

Keep a diary

Keep an exercise diary to record your progress and success. It could also help to identify your barriers to exercise. For example, you may find it difficult to exercise after work if you go home first, so exercise immediately after you leave work before going home. You may also wish to record how you feel. A diary can also be useful in helping you decide when to increase your exercise in terms of frequency, time, and intensity.

Vary your exercise or try a different one

If you become bored with your current activity, try altering it if you can (e.g., taking a different walking/jogging route) or try another activity.

Exercise with others

It can help to exercise with your partner or a friend. You can motivate each other since, having made a commitment to another person, you won't want to let them down. You can also try activities which involve your family, e.g., cycling or swimming.

Wear appropriate clothes

Wear comfortable and appropriate clothes that make you feel good, rather than castoffs.

Provide entertainment

If you exercise alone, use a smartphone to listen to music or books on tape. Be sure to keep one ear open for safety.

Tips to Incorporate Exercise into Your Lifestyle

A healthy lifestyle is an active one. As well as planned exercise (e.g., thirty minutes, three times a week) you should also incorporate activity into your day-to-day life. The following are some ideas to help you incorporate physical activity into your lifestyle.

- Take the stairs instead of lifts/elevators.
- If you work in a large office, walk to talk to your colleagues rather than picking up the phone.
- If you use buses, get off a stop or two earlier and walk.
- Don't worry about finding a parking spot next to the supermarket or shop entrance. By the time you have found one close enough, you could have walked from a further, empty, and less stressful space!
- For small amounts of shopping or other errands, use a bicycle instead of the car, saving you money and the hassle of finding a place to park. If you live in a town or city, you will probably save time, and if you live in the country, you can enjoy the countryside.
- If you have a cordless phone, walk and talk.

How the Doctor Can Help with Your Exercise

You don't always need to see your doctor before you start exercising, but you should make an appointment if:

- You've been diagnosed with heart problems, high blood pressure, or other medical conditions
- You've been sedentary for over a year
- You're over sixty-five and don't currently exercise
- You're pregnant or you're having difficulty getting pregnant
- You have diabetes
- You ever experience chest pains, dizziness, or fainting spells
- You're recovering from an injury or illness
- You have a diagnosed medical condition or illness

Use your best judgment and see your doctor if you have any questions about what you should be doing. Even if you don't have any problems, you may want to get a full checkup before you start exercising, especially if it's been a long time since you've worked out.

Safety Measures

If you want to live a longer, more productive life, you have to exercise most days of the week. You may need to exercise at a lower pace or for shorter periods of time than you did when you were younger. Remember that you may not be able to play hoops to the level of your thirty-year-old colleagues or play as many back-to-back tennis matches as you once could. Make modifications to your routine and play smart. Before you get started, follow these tips so you can avoid injury:

- Get a basic medical screening. Talk with your doctor and find out if you have any conditions that would put you in jeopardy while exercising. If you have a chronic condition that is limiting, you may be able to work out an activity plan within the scope of your ability.
- Find a balanced exercise program and do not rely on one sport to keep you in shape. Follow a program that includes cardiovascular activity, strength training, and stretching.
- Warm up before and cool down after physical activity. Adding a few minutes to your warm-up can make your workouts smoother. Remember that cold muscles are more prone to injury, which is why you are asking for trouble if you skip the warm-up. Try some light jogging or walking as an easy way to warm up.
- Keep it regular. You will not make gains in fitness by cramming your activity into the weekend. Aim for thirty minutes of physical activity every day.
- Take lessons if you can. Hire a trained professional to help you attain and maintain proper form in your sport, even if it is weight training.
- Get the right equipment for your sport. You want to make sure the gear you use for your activity is in good shape and used properly. Think about the condition of your shoes or if you will need a helmet, for example.

- Follow the 10 percent rule. When you are ready to increase your activity level, do so in 10 percent increments. In other words, increase activity by small increments each week. This rule also applies to working with weights.
- Be cautious about adding new exercises. Whether you are a seasoned fitness enthusiast or new to exercise, avoid taking on too many activities at once. It's wisest to add activities gradually.
- Listen to your body and pay attention to the messages your body is sending you. If your knees hurt after you ski, find an easier ski run or maybe think about a different activity that does not hurt your knees.
- Be careful about jumping right back into your routine. Gradually return to your workout routine if you had to take a brief time out because of illness or injury.
- Seek professional help if you injure yourself. Consult your doctor for any injury that is not relieved with home care. Some injuries require medical treatment and will not go away on their own.

Safety Measures to Be Adopted While Running

- Headsets and listening devices make running more pleasant. However, it can also be a distraction, so try keeping one ear clear to listen to your surroundings.
- **Always stay alert and aware of what's going on around you.** The more aware you are, the less vulnerable you are.
- **Carry a cell phone in case you need it for an emergency.**
- **Trust your intuition about a person or an area.** React on your intuition and avoid a person or situation if you're unsure. If something tells you a situation is not "right," it isn't.
- **Alter or vary your running route pattern; run in familiar areas if possible.** In unfamiliar areas, such as

while traveling, contact a local RRCA club or running store. Know where open businesses or stores are located.

- **Run with a partner. Run with a dog**.
- **Write down or leave word of the direction of your run**. Tell friends and family of your favorite running routes.
- **Avoid unpopulated areas, deserted streets, and overgrown trails**. Especially avoid unlit areas at night. Run clear of parked cars or bushes.
- **Carry identification** or write your name, phone number, and blood type on the inside sole of your running shoe. Include any medical information and don't wear jewelry.
- **Ignore verbal harassment**. Use discretion in acknowledging strangers. Look directly at others and be observant, but keep your distance and keep moving.
- **Run against traffic** so you can observe approaching automobiles.
- **Wear reflective material** if you must run before dawn or after dark.
- **Practice memorizing license tags or identifying characteristics of strangers.**
- **Carry a noisemaker** and/or OC (pepper) spray (if it is legal in your state to do so). Get training in self-defense and the use of pepper spray.
- **CALL POLICE IMMEDIATELY** if something happens to you or someone else, or you notice anyone out of the ordinary. It is important to report incidents immediately.

Safety Measures to Be Adopted While Swimming

Swimming is a beneficial way for you to get into shape. Swimming improves endurance, makes the heart muscle stronger, increases circulation, improves muscle strength and flexibility, and helps your body's ability to control and maintain weight. But swimming doesn't come without some risks, such as possible injury and drowning. The Centers for Disease Control and Prevention reports that drowning is the fifth leading cause of accidental death in America [40]. Reduce your risk for injuries and drowning by following a few safety precautions.

Know how to swim

Learning how to swim is one of the best ways to stay safe in the water. If you or other family members don't know how to swim, sign up for beginner swimming courses. Check with your local YMCA and Red Cross center for swimming lessons in your area. Swimming lessons can lessen the risk of drowning among children ages one to four, according to the CDC [40].

Avoid alcohol and drugs

Never swim while under the influence of alcohol or recreational drugs. Alcohol and recreational drugs impair judgment, coordination, and balance, which can be made even worse by outdoor heat and sun exposure. Even if you're a strong swimmer, you can succumb to the effects of alcohol and drugs. If you're taking any medication, ask your doctor about any possible side effects, such as drowsiness or impaired motor skills, and avoid swimming if these medications cause a side effect that would be dangerous to you when in the water.

Lifeguard on duty

If you plan on swimming in a public pool or at a beach, don't enter the water unless a lifeguard is on duty. Even if you're a skilled swimmer, emergencies can happen that are out of your control. Lifeguards are trained for such situations and practice performing rescues and first aid in the event of an emergency. Many public beaches are required to have a lifeguard for every fifty yards of beach.

Supervise children

Approximately one in five people who drown are children fourteen years old and younger, according to the CDC [40]. Closely monitor children even if a lifeguard is present. Make sure that small children wear US Coast Guard-approved life jackets and use flotation devices, but don't rely on flotation devices to replace supervision, warns the American Red Cross [41]. Flotation devices can slip out from underneath a child or deflate, leaving them at risk of drowning. If you need to leave the swimming area, always take your children with you.

Avoid bad weather

Obtain a weather report before swimming. Thunderstorms with strong wind and lightning are dangerous, especially if you're in the water. If the weather report warns of upcoming storms, cancel swimming for that day. If you're swimming and notice lightning or hear thunder, leave the water immediately and seek shelter. Don't return to the water for at least twenty minutes after the last flash of lightning and sound of thunder.

Watch out for rip currents

Even if you're a strong swimmer, rip currents are dangerous and can sweep you out to sea, according to the CDC [42]. Rip currents are caused by waves that move from deep to shallow water. They can pull you into deep water at up to eight feet per second. According to the US Lifesaving Association, more than thirty people drown each year as a result of rip currents [43]. Rip currents can be identified by discolored or choppy water that is filled with debris and traveling away from the shore. Swimming parallel to the shoreline will often free you from a rip current.

Swim within designated areas

Designated swimming areas are marked by ropes or buoys. They're usually clear of rocky underwater terrain, weeds, and other hazards. Motor boats are prohibited from these areas. If you do swim in a river, always bring a swimming buddy with you so you're not alone.

Safety While Lifting Weights

Weight lifting is a great way to increase muscle mass and get in shape, all the while boosting your metabolism. However, there are certain precautions that must be made to avoid injury. Weight-lifting injuries can range from an immediate fracture to chronic aches, pains, and strained ligaments. Pulling a muscle is also a common weight-lifting injury. Here are some useful tips to help you avoid weight-lifting injuries while doing your regular workout:

1. Start Small and Work Your Way Up

Whether you're a bit overconfident about your weight-lifting ability, or you plan on lifting the same amount of weights you did ten years ago in college, lifting weights that are much heavier than you're currently used to is one of the quickest ways to suffer an injury. If it's your first time in the gym, or it has been a while since you last lifted, start off with smaller weights and slowly work your way up to heavier ones. Overexerting yourself by lifting weights that you aren't ready for can lead to severe aches, pains, and strains.

2. Don't Compare Your Weights to Others

One of the biggest mistakes you can make at the gym is trying to secretly compete with someone else who is lifting. While it is important to constantly push yourself to lift more, you don't want to let your ego get in the way of your goals or your overall health, for that matter. Stick to the weights you are comfortable with and slowly work your way up. Don't let the person next to you influence whether you are grabbing eighty pounds when you should be grabbing forty-pounders.

3. Get a Spotter

Having someone to spot you at the gym is important for avoiding weight-lifting injuries. To increase muscle and build strength, you have to constantly push yourself so that you don't plateau. However, lifting more than you are used to can be very dangerous if you are doing it alone. Ask a gym buddy or fellow gym member to spot you whenever you are attempting to lift weights that are well outside your comfort zone.

4. Proper Form

Knowing the proper form for certain weight-lifting exercises is crucial for avoiding injury. Don't be fooled into thinking you understand how a certain exercise works if you've never done it by yourself. If you see someone at the gym performing a certain exercise you'd like to try, just ask for some friendly advice or instructions. Also consider investing in a few sessions with a personal trainer who can instruct you on proper form for exercises you are unfamiliar with.

5. Use the Safety Stoppers

Some fitness equipment comes with catch racks or safety stoppers that can help prevent weight-lifting injuries. A catch rack is a safety device that can be used while doing squatting exercises; the rack will catch the barbell to help prevent getting pinned or throwing out your back. Safety stoppers on certain machines can also be used to prevent heavy weights from falling or crushing you. Make sure you look for such safety devices when attempting to lift heavier weights.

6. Lift in a Slow, Controlled Manner

When pushing yourself to lift heavier or work harder, you may feel tempted to flail about recklessly with the weights you are using. Do not do this. A key to preventing weight-lifting injuries is to not only use proper form, but to lift in a slow, controlled manner. This will also allow you to focus on isolating the muscle you're targeting for the best workout. Sometimes, people get so focused on finishing a repetition or set just for the sake of looking good or to rush through their workout that they aren't even working out their muscles properly. It is always best to take your time when lifting weights.

7. Warm Up

Studies are now showing that stretching before weight lifting is not as beneficial as a good warm-up. Get the blood flowing to the muscles you intend on working by doing the appropriate warm-ups. For example, try doing dynamic warm-up exercises like arm-hugs to loosen your arm and shoulder muscles or knee-highs to help warm up your leg muscles before weight lifting.

8. Wear the Proper Attire

It's surprising to see the number of people who come to the gym and start lifting heavy weights in jeans and flip-flops. Don't be one of these people. Imagine if you were wearing flip-flops, which cause you to lose your footing while weight lifting. Or you could drop a large weight on an exposed toe. For weight lifting, attire is important for safety and comfort, not for style points.

9. Stay Hydrated

Don't become so focused on your workout that you forget to keep yourself properly hydrated. Most of the human body is comprised of water, and when you are weight lifting, you are sweating a lot of that water out. Make sure to always replenish when you get the chance, and even invest in some sports drinks to help with proper hydration and electrolyte balance. Dehydration can lead to a whole other type of weight-lifting injury that can even land you in the hospital.

10. Breathe

One of the most common mistakes for inexperienced weight lifters that can lead to injury is holding their breath. In most cases, you feel tempted to hold your breath at possibly the worst time—when exerting a tremendous amount of effort to complete a rep. Don't cut off your body's oxygen supply when it needs it; make sure you are breathing while you are weight lifting.

Improving Your Exercise— Improve Strength Training

1. Get moving.

For gaining size and lean muscle, focus on four main exercises—squat, bench press, deadlift, and overhead press—which aren't just for powerlifters. Big moves are an invaluable way to increase strength and lean muscle, and there's science to back that up. Research shows that compound moves, such as the squat, recruit multiple muscle groups and elicit a larger hormonal response. This means that these exercises are more effective for building strength and muscle than isolated movements, like the leg extension. As for rep range, doctors often recommend five or fewer repetitions for strength and six to twelve repetitions for gaining size.

2. Be free.

It's not just the moves that matter most; equipment also plays a role. But when it comes to exercise machines, the best advice is to avoid them all. In one study, which compared the performance of free-weight users with the progress of another group using exercise machines, those using free weights outperformed the machine users, showing marked improvement in strength and balance.

3. Carry on.

If size is the goal, it's best to prioritize muscle over miles. That doesn't mean zero cardio, just a different kind. Think about it: a pro football player doesn't train the same way as a world-class endurance athlete. Focus on preserving muscles and burning fat. To accomplish those goals, we recommend using hills sprints and farmer's walks as part of a cardio routine.

4. Eat up.

Packing on muscle usually calls for the consumption of additional calories, but it's important to focus on quality over quantity. According to University of Florida Health, the diet for an athlete or exerciser shouldn't deviate from that of a healthy individual except in the overall amount of food [44]. By avoiding processed foods, refined sugars, and alcohol, and opting for lean protein, complex carbohydrates, and healthy fats, lifters can adequately fuel their body to make gains in the gym.

5. Shut down.

Finding the exercise sweet spot can be a challenge. Too much exercise will result in overtraining, increased risk of injury, and halted progress. On the other hand, too little exercise can make building muscle an uphill battle. It's the combination of work and rest that will lead to results. Creating a training plan that allows for a day off between workouts is one method that can be helpful for beginners. Insufficient sleep can drastically affect performance in the gym and cause a strength-training plateau. Rest is essential to avoid rapid muscle fatigue during subsequent workouts.

Stronger Every Day

There's no secret to making muscles grow. Although the process isn't complicated, it does require commitment and consistency, but by challenging your body on a regular basis and fueling with proper nutrition, results are sure to follow.

Endurance

Increasing your cardiorespiratory endurance and being more active in general not only reduces your risk of developing depression, but also decreases stress and anxiety, increases happiness, self-confidence, and creativity, and improves memory and mental clarity.

Hundreds of studies have been conducted on the effectiveness of exercise in treating clinical depression. A review of 191 studies was published in the journal *Sports Medicine* in 2002 and found considerable support for the value of exercise in reducing depressive symptoms in healthy people and those diagnosed with depression [45]. For mood-boosting benefits, work out at least thirty minutes daily, or more days than not, and look for ways to be more active even when you're not working out.

Some Important Tips:

1. Wake up ten minutes earlier. Then take ten minutes at lunch and ten minutes after work, and you'll easily rake up time for the thirty minutes of daily exercise. Fill the time with a quick workout DVD in the morning, stair climbing in your office building during lunch, and an after-work walk around the parking lot or to a train or bus station past where you typically hop on.

2. Take the magazine test. If you can read a magazine perched on your treadmill screen, you're not working hard enough. Strolling on the treadmill is better than sitting at home eating chips, but high-intensity interval training can deliver the benefits of exercise more efficiently. If you're not working hard enough, increase your running or swimming speed, add an incline on the treadmill, or increase resistance on the elliptical or bike.

3. Use weights on the StairMaster. Combining exercises will maximize your results and help you build cardiorespiratory endurance. Hold a light dumbbell in each hand and either pump your arms to mimic a natural stair-climbing stride or raise the weights above your head and bring them back down as you climb.

4. Jump on the bed. Literally any activity is better than no activity for improving your mood with a release of endorphins. Plus, jumping on the bed can create a sense of nostalgia and reduce stress.

5. Alternate long and hard workouts. Monotonous workouts cause endurance and weight loss to plateau, so increase your cardiorespiratory endurance by alternating between activities that are longer and harder than your regular fitness routine. Begin by incorporating one of the following into your fitness routine each week, then progress to two per week when you feel comfortable.

Long: Jog outside, run on a treadmill, elliptical, cycle, kickbox, row, or swim for at least sixty minutes at a rate where you could simultaneously talk in full sentences.

Hard A: Perform a ten-minute warm-up; fifteen minutes at a comfortably hard aerobic intensity (you shouldn't be able to talk more than a word or two without taking a breath); ten-minute cooldown.

Hard B: Perform a ten-minute warm-up; four to five sets of three minutes of hard exercise, then three minutes active recovery; ten-minute cooldown.

Flexibility

Here is a ten-minute stretching routine for you to do at home. Do these stretches in the prescribed order several times a week after your runs or in the evening when you're in front of the television. The key is never to hold any stretch. Instead, you should move until you feel the resistance, back off immediately, and then repeat.

1. Hamstrings

Getting the hamstrings first is important because they're the gravity-defying muscles that hold up the posterior side of the body. If you're sitting a lot during the day, you're turning those muscles off. Here's what you do:

Lie flat on your back with one leg stretched out in front of you and the other lifted in the air with your knee straight. Keeping your back on the floor, grab onto the raised leg behind the knee (or, if possible, by the calf) and gently pull that leg towards you. You can also use a towel or a band, instead of your bare hands, to facilitate the stretching movement.

2. Adductors

In the adductor stretch, you're bringing the exercising leg away from your midline. The idea here is that you're swinging your leg out and back. So lie on your back with your opposite (nonexercising) leg bent, with that foot flat on the floor (keeping the opposite leg bent takes the extension out of the back). Then bring your other (exercising) leg away from your midline. In this stretch it's best to use a strap or a rope or a towel because it's nice for your outside hand to assist a little bit.

3. Abductors

The outer thigh stretch is a little more intricate, but it's great for people who have lateral hip or IT band issues. Your nonworking leg (your opposite leg) is turned in, and that counterbalances your pelvis. So when you're stretching your right leg, keep your right leg turned out and lead with your right heel. Use your inner leg to cross the midline of your body diagonally.

When you feel resistance, bring the leg down again immediately. That dynamic pumping action really involves the entire length of the muscle and relaxes the tissues.

4. Glutes

This stretch is a crossover with a bent knee. Lie on your back and bring your knee to your opposite shoulder. If you've got back soreness, keep the nonworking leg bent. Otherwise, you can keep the nonworking leg straight and a little bit turned in as a counterbalance for the back. So if you're on your right side, your right hand's on your outer thigh and your left hand's on your outer shin. Bring your knee to your opposite shoulder.

You may want to hold this stretch because it feels so good, but back off as soon as you feel resistance. Be very careful on the first couple of reps because you're resetting those neural pathways and you may have a lot of tension in there. Show your body where you want it to go and you'll see by the third or fourth rep that your body will go way past what you thought it could even do. Do eight to ten reps on one leg, fully unlocking that side, before switching to the other leg.

5. Lower back

Try a bent-knee trunk flexion. Sit on the ground with your knees bent, your legs slightly apart, and your feet flat on the floor. Bring your trunk down, tucking your chin to your chest, so you're getting a full elongation of the back muscles while you use your abdominals to gently go forward. If you've got the range of motion, your hands can assist at your ankles. If your back is extremely tight you could try this exercise from a chair with your feet resting flat on the floor.

Balance

The principle of "if you don't use it, you lose it" definitely applies with balance, particularly as we progress into the vintage realm. The following variations aim to sharpen your nervous system and can be completed anywhere with nothing more than a pillow and/or tennis ball at your disposal. The exercises are listed here sequentially, or in order of difficulty. This way you can move through each level and find the variation that challenges you and progress forward from there. If you can already complete step five, then balance is clearly not an issue for you.

1. Single-Leg Balance: This involves you standing on one leg (for example, the right leg) whilst lifting your left leg upwards and forwards slightly in front of the body. Ensure the right knee is very slightly bent, the hips are square or even, your spine is straight, and your core is engaged at 50 percent of your maximum contraction. Keep the eyes open and look at a consistent spot on the wall in front. In yoga we refer to this as a "drishti," or focus point, that will aid your balance. Hold for sixty seconds, then repeat on the left leg.

2. Single-Leg Balance, Tossing Tennis Ball: As above, except now throw a tennis ball up and across from hand to hand whilst maintaining your "drishti" point. Repeat for sixty seconds.

3. Single-Leg Balance, Standing on Pillow: Fold a standard pillow in half and stand on it to increase instability under your foot. Hold for sixty seconds.

4. Single-Leg Balance, Eyes Shut: As a surfer, when you can hold this for sixty seconds on each individual leg with your eyes shut, it is considered a satisfactory level of balance. As you build up toward sixty seconds, it is advised to stand near a wall so you can touch or hold the wall as required to prevent falling. If this becomes comfortable, you can progress to the next exercise.

5. Single-Leg Balance, Eyes Shut and Standing on Pillow: Sixty seconds.

Setting Goals

Setting process goals is simple, but it's not easy at first for most people. We get distracted. We lose focus. But perfection is a distraction in itself. All that matters is momentum. All that matters is putting one foot in front of the other, millions of times. The cliché "Rome wasn't build in a day" has a meaning that is pertinent to starting an exercise regimen. You simply mustn't be afraid to start. Allow me to expand upon the cliché further. Imagine yourself as the first stonemason to arrive in ancient Rome on the day that the first cobblestone was set in place on a main road. If you were to look around you at the miles of unpaved road winding this way and that and say to yourself, "This is crazy, how am I going to finish this?" you (and perhaps the majority of Western civilization) would fail before you started. The belabored point with respect to starting exercise as a lifestyle is to look at what is in front of you—immediately in front of you. Then proceed. Approach your goals the way that stonemason must have: look at the first stone and the little bit of mortar you have and plop that thing in the dirt. Then, do it again. Not so bad that way, right? Before you know it, Rome has been built!

Here is the path one should follow. The path may change, but the courage it takes to keep moving forward will not.

1. Don't start with "What do I want to do?" but "Who do I want to be?" Describe the kind of person you want to be at the end of this journey, not what you want to achieve. Do you want to be more disciplined, make better health choices, or be a better example for your children?

2. What does that person who you envision do every day? Take that description of the person you want to be and make a list of the kinds of things that person does every day. What are their habits? It helps if you talk to or read up on what people like the person you want to be actually emulate because it's often much less daunting a challenge than you think. For example, Tommy Kono, the only person to hold world records in four classes of Olympic-style weight lifting (and from an era that predates the invention of steroids), only practiced three times a week. He says anyone lifting more than that has a bored coach.

3. Have the courage, the bravery, or the sheer audaciousness to pick ONE of those habits to start with—just one. I can't state this more plainly, and yet everyone chickens out. Pick. One. Habit. ONE. Uno. I know it's not sexy, but it's brave.

4. Ask yourself, "Am I 90 to 100 percent confident that I can do this habit every day for two weeks?" If the answer is no, have the courage to make it smaller. Are you unsure you can go to the gym every day? How about waking up earlier? How about just setting the alarm on your phone? You just need to get started. All that matters is momentum. Rome wasn't built in a day . . . or two, for that matter.

5. Find a trigger, like setting an alarm, you can rely on to remind you. All habits need a trigger or we often just forget. Life gets in the way, so make sure you have something you can't ignore in the way of the status quo. Block your door with your running shoes. Set a recurring six a.m. alarm on your phone. Ask a friend to remind you.

6. Do that habit (or something that makes that habit easier to do) tomorrow, every day. Just show up. Put one foot in front of the other. Even if it's a single step, all that matters is momentum.

7. Track your process. Make a hash mark on your wall. Make a note in your health and fitness website. Tell a stranger on the internet that you put on your running shoes today. You need to see it. You need to celebrate it.

8. Forgive your slipups. It doesn't matter if you miss a day. It doesn't matter if you miss a week. All that matters is momentum, and that means all that matters is today. You have to be obstinate about the present. Have the courage to see your slipups as progress, because the obstacles are on the path. All you have to do is keep moving forward.

The Doctor's Final Remarks
on Nutrition and Exercise

My hope in writing this chapter is that after you have read it, you will feel both inspired and educated as to why nutrition and exercise are essential to health. I am passionate about seeing others succeed. Perhaps it is my past; perhaps it is the memories in my mind of those to whom I wish I might have been able to give just a little knowledge or empowerment to help guide them on their own paths, but I did or could not. Please allow my sentiment and passion to speak to you directly. Take charge of your life; make a difference by improving the quality of your life a little bit each day. You do not have to be a contortionist, gymnast, or professional athlete, or a gain a PhD in nutrition—although you may if you wish—but to appreciate all that life has to offer, you do need to be fit and healthy. And the funny thing is, achieving this is simple. I did not say easy, but it is simple. You literally only need to put one foot forward, followed by another, then pick up the pace and ride on. Throw an apple or two into that mix and you're on your way. Get it? Good!

CHAPTER 10
AGING BY DESIGN

Acquired heart disease develops over time, meaning that aging is a significant risk factor. As we get older, our bodies naturally undergo changes that make us more vulnerable to the risk factors associated with heart disease. As many of my patients often do, it is dangerous to attribute the decline in our physical ability to the aging process and not recognize that this "decline" may be signaling that the heart is under stress. Thus it is important to consider how our bodies change as we age and consider aging by design rather than default.

Driven by a desire to increase longevity, to live a long life, humanity has long sought to overcome nature.

For centuries, we have sought to not only imitate the divine plan, but to interrupt the laws of nature. Thus far, man is partially succeeding along this journey.

Strikingly, many of the advances that have impacted civilization as a whole have occurred in roughly the past hundred years. Within the last twenty of those years, changes in technology and new discoveries have caused sudden, rapid global change at a rate heretofore unseen.

As I've suggested, the majority of this change began around the turn of the twentieth century. Health regulations and public health policies began to focus on improving access to clean water, electricity for refrigeration, pasteurization for dairy processing, and better sewage and garbage disposal. The implementation of these policies was crucial in improving public health in general.

Penicillin was discovered in 1928. Further advances in medical science brought vaccines for smallpox, diphtheria, and polio. Even with two world wars occurring in the first half of the twentieth century, the contributions of science and changes in the social and political landscapes succeeded in shaping advances in public health that resonate to this day.

Has man's quest for longevity yielded any measure of success? Note the following facts [46]:

- In 1925, the average life expectancy at birth was fifty-nine years.
- By 1955, life expectancy increased to seventy years.
- By 1985, life expectancy further increased to seventy-five years.

The gain in life expectancy to seventy-five years in 1985 was due largely in part to early efforts to treat heart disease and curb cigarette smoking. Today, the average life expectancy is nearly eighty years, a full twenty years longer than expected in 1925 [47]. Most of the gains were fueled by further advancements in diagnostics for cancer and heart disease, drug therapy for chronic illnesses, and advances in chemotherapy and radiation treatments for cancer. All of these achievements were accomplished in spite of a raging obesity epidemic. We are now living in an amazing age where there are more people over the age of sixty than under the age of fifteen.

In the words of Dr. King . . .

> Like anybody, I would like to live a long life. Longevity has its place. But I'm not concerned about that now. I just want to do God's will. And He's allowed me to go up to the mountain. And I've looked over. And I've seen the Promised Land. I may not get there with you. But I want you to know tonight, that we, as a people, will get to the Promised Land. And so I'm happy, tonight. I'm not worried about anything. I'm not fearing any man. Mine eyes have seen the glory of the coming of the Lord.
>
> — "I've Been to the Mountaintop"
> Martin Luther King Jr. [48]

As Dr. King lamented, "Longevity has its place," but longevity has created challenges that are just as pervasive as climate change, the flattening global economy, and political upheavals. Quantity of life is not in and of itself a desired goal, or at least, it ought not be; quantity must be accompanied by quality. Longevity, desired by all, can lead to much anxiety within and without. This should come as no surprise as the pace of our gains, an additional twenty years in less than ninety years, outpaces the gains in all of the prior recorded millennia combined. In essence, our culture and our society are unprepared for the spoils of the "divine plan."

We live in a society built for young people. Institutions such as transportation systems, parks and recreation, educational systems, and real estate subdivisions with single-family homes are largely built for younger, stronger, more vital populations. The needs of our elder populations are, in general, an afterthought.

With our population living longer lives, we must consider that the concept of useful work beyond the age of sixty will one day become commonplace. Businesses should rethink the notion that a younger workforce is a more productive workforce. That thinking should be transformed into the conceptualization that an older, more settled, mature, and experienced worker can and will be just as productive if not more productive than a younger, less committed one. There exists in those who have honed their skills over time a wisdom and insight that only maturity and experience can bring. As a society, we must recognize and utilize these talents.

Aging by Design

If we are likely to live longer, we are going to need to apply some forethought as to how we achieve quality of life in these later years . . . hence, Aging by Design.

As sudden as aging may seem, no one wakes up one day and suddenly finds that they are in a ninety-year-old body. If you know what's in store, you can plan ahead and take a bit of time early in life to think about later in life. The good news: if you feel like you are already there, then no need to worry, for it is never too late to live well.

Here's a Body Timeline:

Age 18. The collagen and elastin content of the skin begin to decline by 1 percent per year [49]. Slow it down by eating well, exercising, and avoiding smoking and excessive exposure to UV light. UV light rays are not exclusive to the sun; some lightbulbs contain this type of radiation.

Age 30. Lung function declines by 1 percent per year after you turn twenty-five [50]. Again, don't smoke. The antidote to decreasing lung function is exercise. Stay cardiovascularly fit, and you will be more likely to maintain lung function for much longer.

Age 35. Bone mass begins to decline. This process is faster in women after menopause. The antidote: exercise and diet. Eat a wide variety of healthy foods and perform mild to moderate weight-bearing exercises. You will likely beat the odds.

Age 40. Muscle loss begins and fat increases. Exercise is the antidote. Sense a recurring theme here?

Age 45. Sight begins to decline. There is an association between smoking and UV light exposure to the development of a number of diseases that affect the eyes. The solution here is to wear sunglasses with UV protection and to not smoke. Other ways to keep your eyes healthy are:

- A diet rich in antioxidants (such as fruit and vegetables)
- Keeping blood-sugar levels within normal limits (if you are a diabetic, you'll want to keep what is known as "tight glycemic control")
- Keep lipid levels and total cholesterol within normal limits
- Maintain a healthy body weight
- Keep blood pressure within normal limits

Age 50. Now the stuff you can't see or feel begins to decline, like the kidneys. Remind yourself as you exercise to maintain good fluid balance. Don't get dehydrated.

Age 60. The gastrointestinal tract loses nutrient-absorbing capacity. Therefore, a vitamin may become necessary. Also, hearing loss begins naturally at age sixty. Avoid loud noises and wear ear protection if you work or play in noisy environments.

Age 65. Heart disease begins to kick in. And you know the antidote already. All together now: Yes, exercise. Also—eat right and don't smoke.

Age 70. Brain changes and cognitive decline can speed up, so stay active. What is our magic word of the day? You guessed it, EXERCISE. But not just physical exercise; mental exercise is just as important to brain health. Stay engaged in meaningful, thought-provoking activities.

Age Disrupters

Yes, as you might imagine, we are not the only ones seeking the "divine plan." Scientists and drug companies are also hard at work looking for a solution to slow the aging process. At the University of Texas Health Sciences Center in San Antonio, Texas, there is a mouse named UT2598 that is on track to becoming the oldest mouse to ever live. Those darn mice live about 2.3 years on average, and UT is now 3 years old [51]. The oldest recorded mouse lived for four years [52].

According to researchers studying UT, he is lean, mean, and active. UT is being fed a compound called rapamycin, a drug used to prevent organ rejection in transplant patients. This is just one example of a number of investigational studies underway around the world aimed at unlocking the mystery of aging in biological and physical structures and interrupting that process with a medication.

Of course, we know that our environment and lifestyle are the major players in the development of most diseases, including cancer, heart disease, immune disorders, and brain degeneration. However, the aging process is a factor that increases susceptibility to disease as body systems and processes lose peak functionality. Locating a potential panacea or at least something to delay the onset of age-related changes would be a blessing, to say the least.

Rapamycin, an antibiotic, was discovered in 1964 from dirt samples recovered from Easter Island. It even seems to work on older mice. Now, I know what you might be thinking. Not so fast, my friends. As it turns out, rapamycin interrupts the function of a gene called mTOR found in both mice and men. The gene mTOR acts as a sort of traffic signal for how cells take in and use energy. In the presence of abundant food supply for cells, it tells them to continue to grow. When food is not plentiful, it quiets the cells. The more active cells seem to age faster. Thus, rapamycin slows down mTOR, which in turn slows down the cellular activity.

So my friends, what does this sound like? Yes, you guessed it: stop eating too much and exercise.

Although UT is lean and mean at 30 percent less weight than his counterparts, he is at higher risk of developing cataracts and diabetes as observed in other mice treated with the drug. Male mice also tend to experience gradual loss of testicular function, which is not exactly a selling point for longevity gurus. Very few things come without a price in medicine.

Other anti-aging research is focused on gene therapy, targeting telomeres, which seem to act as DNA-stabilizing products. As DNA divides with cells, telomeres signal the end of this process and eventually disappear altogether. Telomerase, an enzyme that helps lengthen telomeres, is the target of this research. Finding a way to increase telomerase activity to lengthen telomeres and thus diminish cellular decline is the hopeful goal of this research.

Get Your Head in the Game

The great divide between mind, body, and soul is no longer a divide. The notion that the mind is home to the abstract and the ethereal and the body home to the mishmash of mechanics and biology is no longer sound thinking. Research has firmly established that one's moods, feelings, and thoughts powerfully influence physiology and the inner workings of our bodies. The old saying "you are only as old as you feel" may soon be "you are only as old as you choose to be." The research is mounting to support the premise that your outlook, personality, and optimism have a profound impact not just on how you feel, but on how your cells age.

A plethora of studies have shown that meditation can downregulate a gene that codes for production of inflammatory cells. Remember the telomeres we discussed earlier. As it turns out, these are much shorter in people with depression and highly stressful lives. If that's not enough to get your attention, in one study on newborn cord blood samples, telomeres were shorter in babies born to mothers under stress. The more stress, the shorter the telomeres [53].

Can you guess what else might lengthen telomeres and reduce stress in addition to meditation and cognitive behavioral therapy? You guessed it! Exercise.

What about brain games? Yes, they help to stimulate the mind and keep the mind active. But you don't need Lumosity (a program that provides various brain games) to stimulate your mind. There are plenty of good, wholesome, positive activities for seniors that are free or very inexpensive. The classic crossword puzzle of my mother's generation is still around, and along with reading and journaling, these are all excellent means of engaging and activating the brain.

Nutrition and Diet

Let me say for starters, my biggest concern with our nutritional state in this country is volume. We simply eat too much. I remember growing up and buying a coke in an eight-ounce glass bottle. They are now collector's items. I remember the small bags of potato chips for sale as a single item. Now, those bags are sold as multipacks, and only the big grabs on the shelf are a single item.

Our thinking about diets should change, and the focus should not be on the often-advertised short-term gains, but on sustaining a healthier life. We should carefully choose foods that will support the nutrition our bodies require. Furthermore, we should think about disease prevention and avoiding foods that contribute to disease development.

The bottom line is to lower the volume, increase fruit and vegetable content, limit red and animal-based meats, and avoid fried and processed foods. Be wary of sugar supplements, refined sugars, and artificial sweeteners.

A Well-Planned Life

As my dad would say: "Don't be in a rush to DO, but plan to DO for a mighty long time!" Embrace a lifestyle that seeks to maximize your quality of living. That means a largely plant-based diet, daily exercise—including other stress management techniques such as yoga and meditation—and a social support network. In summary, eat well (but not too much), move more, stress less, and love more. In the words of the great Persian poet Omar Khayyam,

> The Moving Finger writes; and, having writ,
> Moves on: nor all thy Piety nor Wit
> Shall lure it back to cancel half a line,
> Nor all thy Tears wash out one Word of it.

CHAPTER 11
CRITICAL
HEALTH-CARE
COMMUNICATION

I can bore you with the many definitions of communication, but this would be missing the mark. Instead, I will reiterate my goal in writing this book, which is to impart to you the life-saving necessity of communicating what you are experiencing with loved ones and health-care providers. If there is one thing that you should take from this book, let it be that when you feel something unusual—tell someone.

What Is Communication?

It is common sense to consider the fact that communication requires both a sender and a receiver in order to be successful. What is less common is the understanding that communication is directly affected by the way in which the transmission occurs, as well as by the ritual aspects of communication. Transmission of an idea must be done with great care. It is very easy to confuse even the simplest of messages when attempting to explain it to another person. There are many reasons for this, some of which involve not only the content of the message itself, but the tone of the sender's message or the nonverbal cues projected by the sender. The receiver of the message also plays a part in achieving accurate communication. A receiver may misinterpret the message by interpreting a different meaning from the sender's tone than that intended. Also physical, nonverbal cues given off by the sender may be interpreted incorrectly by the receiver. These are just some of the things that can go wrong during the transmission stage of communicating.

The ritual aspects of communication also have a role in the quality of the message sent and received. Ritual aspects of communication include the formal and informal parts of a message. For example, people typically address the receiver by name before beginning a conversation instead of saying "hey," unless the sender has an intimate and informal style established with the receiver. Social position also influences the way in which communication occurs. For an extreme example, consider having a conversation between the "normal, average Joe" and the president of the United States. In most people, during a sit-down with a president there would be a natural tendency to defer or agree with most statements during such a two-way conversation. One would not typically feel comfortable arguing openly and speaking casually to the president.

These are just a few examples of how both the transmission and the ritual aspects of any communication must be understood and examined by both parties in order to be effective. So, how does all of this apply to your communication with your family or with your doctor?

Why Is Quality Communication with Your Physician Important?

The Interview: When your doctor sits with you to interview you about a problem that you are having, he or she is in the process of developing a diagnosis based on what you communicate to him. It is during this interview that most decisions about what might be affecting you are made. Therefore, the quality of the interview becomes a critical component of your physician's ability to provide an accurate diagnosis. Interruptions, the physician's temperament, the patient's presentation of data, personal feelings of both parties about one another, and many other issues directly impact the quality of the interview. It is at this portion of a physician visit that understanding communication can help you deliver a message that is received appropriately.

Follow These Tips to Get through an Interview Successfully:

- Bring a list of your symptoms to the meeting.
- Read directly from the list (including times, dates, and circumstances).
- Be brief and to the point with your presentation.
- If you are unable to write or read a list for some physical or emotional reason, bring someone with you who can.
- Do not be dismissed. Make sure that you are heard. To be fair to the physician, however, make sure that you can deliver this presentation in a reasonable amount of time, say, three to five minutes.
- If you find resistance to what you are trying to accomplish, say the following: "I realize that you are very busy. I have carefully recorded my findings that I need you to hear. This is extremely important to me and will take only a few minutes."

Doing these things should see you through your meeting with your doctor. Keep in mind that most doctors today are very busy, so give them the respect that they deserve for their time while at the same time pleasantly demanding that you be heard. You deserve airtime, as your health is the issue during any physician visit. Applying these techniques will help you achieve effective communication and mutual respect.

Compliance: The patient's role in successful treatment of their health concerns is paramount. You, as the patient, have a responsibility to follow the physician's treatment plan to the letter. The relationship between physician and patient ought to be one of mutual trust, and communication is the way to build this trust. Ideally, if you have successfully communicated your part of your symptomology to your doctor and if your doctor has heard you clearly, you will likely have a diagnosis and treatment plan based on sound information. This is why you now have an obligation to act in accordance with that treatment plan.

However, should you disagree with the treatment plan, it is your responsibility to explain this directly to your doctor. This may be a very uncomfortable conversation, since there is an unspoken ritual aspect to this relationship that involves the doctor being highly educated in these areas and the patient (more often than not) not having the same access to information. This phenomenon has the ability to sometimes cause a patient to feel inferior or unable to question a treatment plan or diagnosis. Nothing could be further from reality. You, as the patient, have the right to understand your diagnosis or treatment plan. In the end, if you are unable to get a satisfactory explanation as to why a certain plan or diagnosis is being proposed, you have the right to change your physician or get a second opinion.

Steps to Take to Build Compliance with Treatment:

- If you disagree with your doctor, say so.
- If the cost of medication or other services are such that you cannot follow the plan, say so.
- If you do not understand instructions given to you, say so.
- If you have beliefs or cultural practices that make compliance with a treatment plan impossible, speak up.

There is a common thread with building compliance and trust with your physician. That common thread is communication. You simply must take the time and gather the courage to speak up on your own behalf, or alternatively, find someone you trust who can accompany you and help you achieve this goal.

Why Worry about Good Communication?

This one is easy. Adverse events (problems that occur that are potentially harmful to patients) are largely due to human error. This error is poor communication. While you do not have control over how other staff members in a physician's office communicate, or over how your physician communicates, you do have control over how you communicate. This power is not a small thing. By taking the time to clearly let your doctor in on what is happening, you are far more likely to get a positive result.

Miscommunications to Remember

Even a small error can have calamitous results. Let's say, for example, that a patient feels intimidated by their doctor because this physician has an elevated manner of speech, a habit of not looking the patient in the eye, and spends only two minutes with the patient during visits. Making matters worse, let's say that the patient in question did not finish high school and feels unable to explain what he is experiencing to the doctor because of his inability to speak at the physician's level of expression. This patient, then, enters the office each visit with the full intent of explaining how on many mornings and often during the middle of the night he wakes up with intense pain in his chest. Knowing he shouldn't be eating fried foods at all, particularly before going to bed, he feels embarrassed about revealing this information, as this could be the cause of the pain. But the pain is very bad and sometimes lasts for many hours, making it difficult to sleep. He realizes that he should inform the physician. However, each time he sits down with the physician, he notes that the doctor simply does not appear interested. He decides to not tell his story and to just "live with the pain." Weeks later, he is hospitalized with a major heart attack that has done permanent damage to the heart muscle.

Does this story seem farfetched? I will tell you that it is not. There are many patients who have felt the same or similarly and did not speak up. Their symptoms, although severe, go unnoticed, often with severe and avoidable results.

Communicating one's needs and experiences are the basis for the physician-patient relationship. Essential to the success of this interaction is an understanding on the part of both parties as to the importance of communicating effectively and how to do so. Control over communication lies in the hands of the patient, since controlling oneself is the only option. Taking the time to understand your physician and his or her strengths, weaknesses, and obstacles to communication is a must. It is also equally important to work on the delivery of the message to the physician. Clarity, brevity, and, when necessary, insistence on being heard are all strategies that, when used by a patient, can mean the difference between life and death.

CHAPTER 12
WHAT TO DO WHEN
HEART ATTACK
HITS YOU

Face it, no matter how much or how little we do to prevent it, no matter how much exercise, diet, or denial we experience, most of us fear on some level the thought of having a heart attack. Many have known someone who has suffered from a heart attack, and there is a universal, primal image of a person clutching their chest that can be conjured up when the phrase "heart attack" comes to mind. So, with so much energy being spent to avoid this phenomenon, what do you do if or when it happens to you?

In the First Moments:
When You Think You Are Having a Heart Attack

You are eating breakfast alone in your home, your husband is at work, your kids are off to school, and you are following the typical morning ritual before getting off to work yourself. You woke up early this morning with a strong feeling of heartburn, tried to go back to sleep, but could not. Heartburn is not that unusual for you, but this bout was particularly strong and lasted about an hour. The feelings seemed to subside after that, still present but not overwhelming.

While reaching in the overhead cabinet for coffee, you feel a slight numbness in your left arm. You also note a feeling of being tired, of general fatigue. It is early in the morning and you did not sleep well, which might explain your feeling tired, and the feeling in your arm is not painful, just an odd feeling (so you ignore that as well). Getting ready, you go upstairs to take a shower.

On the way up the stairs, you begin to feel slightly short of breath—nothing dramatic, but nevertheless short of breath. You've not been exercising lately, so perhaps this is related to not being physically fit.

This story is not unusual. The picture presented here is of a busy individual on their way to work who may be experiencing the first signs and symptoms of a heart attack. Rationalization of these signs and symptoms are common, largely because we don't have time to overreact (or are worried about being perceived as overreacting) to a situation. The person described here may in fact not be experiencing a heart attack. Alternatively, these signs and symptoms may be the first in a series that become progressively more severe, resulting ultimately in a heart attack.

Communication of this experience is the first step, one that is all too often overlooked by people in this exact situation. What you need to realize and remember is that time equals heart muscle. In the setting of a real heart attack, where muscle is being deprived of oxygen, muscle tissue is dying. It is possible to delay or even prevent the death of tissue if prompt intervention occurs. The solution is to present these signs and symptoms to a health-care provider immediately. Call your doctor. Call an ambulance. Communicate your experience clearly to these individuals. Time equals muscle.

Below you will find steps that you need to be aware of in order to properly address what could be a heart attack. Please learn them, and even if you only THINK you are experiencing them, call a health-care provider.

1. Know the Warning Signs of a Heart Attack
- Chest pain, tightness, pressure, squeezing, fullness, stabbing

- Discomfort in the upper body: one or both arms, the back, neck, jaw, or stomach
- Difficulty breathing; may be with or without chest discomfort
- A pounding heart, or changes in rhythm of heart
- Heartburn, vomiting, nausea, pain in the stomach area
- Cold sweats
- Dizziness or feeling lightheaded

Women May Feel Slightly Different, and More Commonly Feel the Following:
- Sudden difficulty breathing, vomiting, nausea, indigestion, sleepiness, feeling achy
- Feeling illness (no chest pain)
- Strange feeling or slight pain in back, chest, neck, jaw, arms (no chest pain)
- Difficulty sleeping
- Feeling anxious

2. Time is Muscle

If the above symptoms occur for longer than a few minutes, and you feel a strong sense of feeling very ill and in a way that you never have before when you've felt indigestion, severe stress, or anxiety . . . GET MEDICAL HELP IMMEDIATELY. Call 911.

3. Do Not Drive Yourself to the Hospital

The ambulance has equipment and medical devices and medications that you do not. They also have healthy and experienced personnel who can assist you through these crucial first moments of experiencing symptoms. Oxygen, pain medications and aspirin, equipment to assist breathing, and an EKG can be performed while en route to the hospital. This information will be presented to hospital staff and referred to a cardiologist so that immediate action can be taken at the hospital upon your arrival. If you need to have stenting or an angioplasty, the staff needed and rooms to perform these interventions can be made ready for you so that you get the help you need immediately.

Driving yourself to the hospital is never an option. Not only would you miss the opportunity to get appropriate care quickly while underway, but you may be so ill (or become so ill) that you are unable to reach your destination. Many a person has set out for the hospital, pulled over to the side of the road due to the pain, and been unable to reach for the phone because of the pain. In these cases, that last moment is often the end of the story. Alternatively, you may lose consciousness or become dizzy as symptoms progress, becoming a hazard to others on the road.

4. Communicate

When you call 911, or whomever you speak to, tell them, "I think I'm having a heart attack." If able, notify them of your address and maintain communication if possible. This is all that you need to do. This phrase will put into action a team of individuals uniquely prepared to see you through a heart attack.

5. Aspirin

Chew one uncoated aspirin. Don't worry about water or anything else. Simply bite down and chew. It will not taste pleasant, but it just may reduce the formation of blood clots that can cause heart attack (or worsen already existing damage).

6. Advocate for Yourself

If you believe that you are not feeling right, do not let anyone tell you differently. You will likely know the difference between indigestion or anxiety and a heart attack (even though they may seem similar at certain stages). If someone, anyone, tells you that they don't think you are having one, be sure that they've performed a thorough cardiac examination to determine otherwise. This includes an EKG, laboratory work, and ideally seeing or knowing that a cardiologist has seen your EKG. In the emergency room, depending upon the time of day or where you live, it is not unusual for a cardiologist to receive an EKG at his or her home to make the initial evaluation of what is happening with your heart.

You've Just Survived a Heart Attack. Now What?

Don't change much—only everything

You've done everything right. You've received immediate care during the first signs and symptoms, have been hospitalized and received the appropriate treatment, and are now in the recovery phase of your illness. Where do you go from here? What actions do you take, and what can be expected? Well, we've discussed the lifestyle changes you will need to undertake: diet, exercise, medication regimen aimed at risk reduction and optimizing the performance of the heart, and stress reduction chief among them. You can also expect to go through some amount of additional testing (cardiac catheterizations, stress testing, etc.) to determine how your heart is performing after your recovery period to determine the amount of damage to your heart as well as to assess your coronary arteries.

How long is recovery?

Base your activity level on your doctor's recommendation. But, in general, it is a very good idea to get and stay socially and physically involved in activities as your condition permits. Sleep is also extremely important; you should get a complete eight hours of sleep each night as well as a nap, if necessary, during your recovery period. The specific length of time that recovery takes will vary for everyone, but you should be active as much as your body allows as a general rule of thumb. Again, check with your doctor or health-care provider for the final word on the exact amount of activity that you should be engaging in.

Working

Anywhere from two weeks to three months is a good general range of time to recover before returning to work. There are certain types of work environments or duties that may no longer be acceptable after a heart attack. Work with your doctor to determine whether or not you can continue with the same type of employment in which you were engaged prior to your heart attack.

Depression

Emotions commonly run high for at least six months after a heart attack. Typically, survivors may feel depression along with anger and fear. Many people feel resentment, asking themselves, "Why me?" in response to such an event. Often people feel extreme anxiety with any pain that reminds them of the heart attack, thinking, "Am I going to die?" as the events of previous experience are relived. This is extremely common, and it is important for both patients and loved ones to react with some patience and understanding when dealing with these emotions. Also, there are support groups as well as other sources of help available (such as individual therapy) for heart-attack survivors. It is important to surround yourself with a strong, competent team of health-care professionals and family and friends who will help make your recovery period a less bumpy ride.

Chest pain . . . again?

Angina pectoris or unstable angina is a condition in which a person has persistent chest pain as a result of previous damage to the heart (in the time immediately following a heart attack, for example). This is a common condition after a heart attack, which you may or may not experience. If you do experience this condition, it should feel like light pain or pressure in the chest area that happens during exercise, a heavy meal, or an emotional event. This feeling should subside after several minutes. If, however, it does not subside, seek medical attention immediately, as there is a possibility that this may be another heart attack. Call 911 or speak to a health-care provider immediately.

Cardiac rehabilitation

Getting into a cardiac rehabilitation program is also extremely helpful. These programs are run by a team of health-care professionals under medical supervision. They will teach you directly how to adapt to your current situation by engaging you in supportive lifestyle activities and changes. The benefit of this kind of therapy cannot be overstated. You will likely experience emotions and difficulties that you had not anticipated, and these programs are designed to deal with them. If cardiac rehab is something that is available to you, please indulge yourself.

Lifestyle Changes—The Big Ones

We have spent a fair amount of time in previous chapters reviewing risks to the heart and preventative measures that can be taken to avoid complications. But, after you've experienced a heart attack, you are now more likely to have another, and having a new lease on life, so to speak, may be sufficient motivation to prevent a second one. These are the big changes that need to be made after having a heart attack:

- **Stop Smoking** and stay away from smokers. This is a tough one, but have you heard the expression "if you go to the barber shop enough times, you probably will end up with a haircut?" It's very true; staying away from smokers can help you stay away from taking up smoking. The reverse is unfortunately also true.

- **Increase Activity.** Get regular physical activity to control depression, lower weight and cholesterol levels, and keep your blood pressure under control.
- **Eat Well.** Weight, blood pressure, and cholesterol levels can all be lowered with proper nutrition. Take the time to do these things well.

In the final analysis, surviving a heart attack is a combination of the recognition of signs and symptoms followed by early intervention. From that point onward, surviving a heart attack means including important changes in your lifestyle. Also, developing an awareness of emotions and how they are affecting you and your family can be very helpful in making recovery successful. With a little help and a lot of work you will be well on your way through recovery and adapting to life after a heart attack. One last note of encouragement—remember that it is never too late to try. Where there is hope, there is strength. Find hope, and you will find the strength to thrive.

APPENDIX

Medications and Complementary Treatments Used in Heart Disease

Please use the appendix below to guide your understanding of the common medications and therapies used to treat heart disease.

Angiotensin-Converting-Enzyme Inhibitors (also called ACE inhibitors)

One type is ACE inhibitors. ACE stands for angiotensin-converting enzyme. Angiotensin is a naturally occurring substance in the body that constricts (tightens) blood vessels, causing blood pressure to elevate. ACE inhibitors decrease the effectiveness of angiotensin, causing the blood vessels to relax, which in turn reduces blood pressure. ACE inhibitors are also used after a heart attack or in the case of heart failure (poor pumping action), diabetes (ACE inhibitors do not negatively affect blood sugar), kidney disease (help control protein in the urine), or lung disease (do not affect asthma or COPD flare-ups).

Examples of ACE Inhibitors Include:

- Vasotec (enalapril)
- Accupril (quinapril)
- Altace (ramipril)
- Zestril (lisinopril)
- Capoten (captopril)

Common side effects of ACE inhibitors:

- Cough
- Dizziness
- Headache
- High potassium (leading to irregular heartbeat)
- Swelling of legs
- Rash
- Fever

Angiotensin Receptor Blockers or ARBs:

ARBs are similar to ACE inhibitors as they affect the action of angiotensin on blood vessels. By blocking the binding of angiotensin to blood vessels, they prevent vasoconstriction and therefore lower blood pressure. Thus, these medications are another option for treating high blood pressure. Similar to ACE inhibitors in action, they are also commonly used in patients who cannot tolerate ACE inhibitors and in cases of heart failure (poor pumping of the heart).

Some examples:
- Atacand (candesartan)
- Avapro (irbesartan)
- Cozaar (losartan)
- Benicar (olmesartan)
- Diovan (valsartan)

Some common side effects of ARBs:
- Cough
- Dizziness
- Headache
- High potassium (leading to irregular heartbeat)
- Swelling of legs
- Rash
- Fever

Beta Blockers

Beta blockers block beta receptors, which are responsible for the stimulatory effects of adrenaline. Adrenaline causes an increase in heart rate and blood pressure by constricting blood vessels. Therefore, through their action, beta blockers lower heart rate and blood pressure. Many times beta blockers are used in combination with diuretics, or "water pills."

Examples of beta blockers include:
- Tenormin (atenolol)
- Lopressor (metoprolol)
- Toprol (metoprolol)
- Coreg (carvedilol)
- Inderal (propanolol)

Some common side effects of beta blockers:
- Slow heartbeat
- Dizziness
- Fatigue
- Shortness of breath (asthma, COPD)
- Leg swelling
- Erectile dysfunction

Diuretics (Water Pills)

Diuretics reduce the amount of water (fluid) inside the blood vessels. It is easiest to explain how diuretics work by thinking of our vascular system as a water tank: the more water in the tank, the higher the pressure. Water pills help lower the amount of water in the tank and thus lower the pressure inside. In addition, as blood moves through our arteries and veins, the lower volume created by lowering the tank decreases resistance to flow and thus reduces blood pressure.

Examples of diuretics:
- Lasix (furosemide)
- Aldactone (spironolactone)
- Dyazide (triamterene)

- Diuril (chlorothiazide)
- Different combinations of hydrochlorothiazide (HCTZ)

Common side effects:
- Excessive urination (they are supposed to make you urinate)
- Low potassium; some cause high potassium
- High potassium; some cause low potassium
- Dehydration
- Dry mouth
- Irregular heartbeat (potassium)
- Kidney failure
- Thirst

Alpha Blockers

This brings us to another type of heart medication called alpha blockers. Alpha receptors are responsible for constricting the peripheral arteries. Remember, when there is constriction in a blood vessel, the blood pressure increases. Alpha receptors in the smooth muscle of the peripheral arteries are blocked by these medications. This causes the peripheral arteries to dilate, or relax, thus causing the blood pressure to be lowered. These medications work very similarly to the beta blockers, except that they work on a different type of receptor, the alpha receptor.

Examples of alpha blockers:
- Hytrin (terazosin)
- Cardura (doxazosin)
- Flomax (tamsulosin)
- Uroxatral (alfuzosin)

Some common side effects of alpha blockers:
- Dizziness
- Fast heartbeat
- Swelling
- Fatigue

Calcium Channel Blockers

Calcium channel blockers restrict the movement of calcium into the cytoplasm (inside) of the muscle cells of the heart. Calcium is one of the minerals required for the heart to contract. With this reduction of calcium, the heart cannot pump as forcefully, thus reducing the pressure of the blood that is pumped out. It's kind of like taking a V-8 engine out of a car and putting in a four-cylinder engine—not quite as powerful.

Examples of calcium channel blockers:
- Norvasc (amlodipine)
- Procardia (nifedipine)
- Adalat (nifedipine)
- Calan (verapamil)
- Covera (verapamil)
- Cardizem (diltiazem)

Common side effects of calcium channel blockers:
- Leg swelling
- Increased blood sugar
- Increased blood cholesterol
- Slow heartbeat
- Fast heartbeat
- Constipation

Antiplatelet Agents/Thrombin Inhibitors

Platelets are tiny cells in our vascular system that promote blood clotting. They do this by combining with a protein in our blood called thrombin. Through various mechanisms, antiplatelet agents block the effect of platelets, therefore promoting smoother blood flow and a lower likelihood of clot formation within arteries. When clots occur in the vascular system, they can lead to heart attacks and strokes, among other things.

These medications are an important adjunct to stenting of blood vessels, in particular blood vessels of the heart (coronary arteries). Therefore, after a stenting procedure, your doctor will generally prescribe these types of medications for an extended period of time. Unlike some of the other common heart medications, these drugs can be particularly dangerous if you are undergoing a surgical procedure, including heart surgery, as they can lead to life-threatening bleeding complications during or after the surgical procedure. Be sure to always inform your doctor of **ALL** medications you are taking.

Examples of antiplatelet agents/thrombin inhibitors:
- Aspirin
- Plavix (clopidogrel)
- Xarelto (rivaroxaban)
- Effient (prasugrel)
- Pradaxa (dabigatran)

Common side effects of these agents:
- Bruising
- Bleeding (from just about anywhere, including stomach, colon, brain, urine, etc.)
- Fatigue
- Rash

Blood Thinners (Also Called Anticoagulants)
Unlike antiplatelet and antithrombin, agents that work **indirectly** by blocking the action of platelets and thrombin, these drugs are used to **directly** block the body's clotting cascade at various points along the clotting pathway. The net effect is to prevent blood clots within the vascular system. These drugs are used to treat various clotting defects related to atrial fibrillation (irregular beating of the atrium) and deep venous thrombosis (DVT) to prevent clots on heart valves and stents and after certain heart attacks and strokes.

Examples include:
- Coumadin (warfarin)
- Lovenox (enoxaparin)

- Argatroban (injection only)
- Heparin (injectable—through veins that are below skin, NOT by mouth)

Common side effects:
- BLEEDING from anywhere
- Skin rash
- Allergy to platelets (called HIT, generally related to heparin)
- Low platelet count

Antianginals (for Chest Pain Relief)

Nitroglycerin (NTG) is commonly used when a heart attack is suspected. It works by dilating blood vessels, which allows blood to flow more freely through the heart. It is administered by mouth, below the tongue (for fast action), or through the veins. The most common side effects include low blood pressure (hypotension) and headache.

Renexa (ranolazine) is a newer medication used to treat chest pain that is refractory to standard treatment with NTG and calcium channel blockers. It works by altering the opening of sodium and potassium channels on the cells of heart muscles. Common side effects include dizziness, headache, nausea, and abnormal heartbeat (prolonged QTC interval, which is detected by EKG).

Calcium channel blockers can also be used to treat chest pain.

Statins

Statins are a class of medicines that are frequently used to lower blood-cholesterol levels. The drugs act by blocking the action of a chemical produced in the liver calle HMG-CoA reductase, thereby reducing production of cholesterol. Although cholesterol is necessary for normal function of cells, overproduction and high levels can contribute to the development of atherosclerosis (plaques) within arteries. As these plaques build up within the artery, they can lead to reduced blood flow, which may cause chest pain (angina), or they may rupture and lead to a heart attack. In the brain, these same two processes can lead to stroke. By reducing blood-cholesterol levels and thus its availability to increase plaque buildup, statins lower the risk of chest pain (angina), heart attack, and stroke.

Complementary Treatments

Fiber

Although weight loss combined with lower intake of dietary forms of fat have the greatest impact on lowering LDLs (recall that these are lipids that contribute to coronary artery disease and other conditions), fiber is thought to also be beneficial in lowering LDLs. The type of fiber matters, though; you want to focus your attention on vegetables, fruits, oats, and barley. These are quality sources of fiber that, when ingested at twenty-five to thirty grams per day, may help lower overall LDL levels. The effect of all of this lipid lowering may be to help prevent heart disease or potentially to decrease the negative effects of LDLs in the blood.

Vitamins

Current research suggests acquiring vitamins through food rather than supplementation when attempting to have a positive effect on heart-disease-related concerns. The big vitamins with respect to the heart to increase intake of are vitamin E and beta carotene. Vitamin E may be found in green leafy vegetables, papaya, nuts, seeds, legumes, as well as whole grains. Beta carotene is found in most dark orange, dark green, and red fruits and vegetables.

REFERENCES

1. Alwan, A., Dr. (2011). "Burden: Mortality, morbidity and risk factors." In *Global status report on noncommunicable diseases 2010*. Geneva, Switzerland: World Health Organization.
2. "Heart Disease Fact Sheet." (2015, November 30). Retrieved from http://www.cdc.gov/dhdsp/data_statistics/fact_sheets/fs_heart_disease.htm.
3. US DHHS, CDC, & NCHS (n.d.). "About Underlying Cause of Death, 1999–2014." Retrieved from http://wonder.cdc.gov/ucd-icd10.html.
4. CDC Newsroom. "Press Release." (2013, May 2). Retrieved from https://www.cdc.gov/media/releases/2013/p0502-physical-activity.html.
5. "Chronic Disease Overview." (2016, February 23). Retrieved from http://www.cdc.gov/chronicdisease/overview/index.htm.
6. Thurman, H. (1972). *The Creative Encounter*. Richmond, IN: Friends United Press.
7. "New Lifetime Poll Shows More than Half of Women Know Heart Disease is their Number One Killer, Yet Only One in Three Believe they are Personally at Risk." (2006, February 2). Retrieved from http://www.prnewswire.com/news-releases/new-lifetime-poll-shows-more-than-half-of-women-know-heart-disease-is-their-number-one-killer-yet-only-one-in-three-believe-they-are-personally-at-risk-55178357.html.

8. "Only One In Three Women Believe They Are Personally At Risk For Heart Disease." (2012, May). Retrieved from http://www.nhlbi.nih.gov/health/educational/hearttruth/about/risk-awareness.htm.

9. "How Does Heart Disease Affect Women?" (n.d.). Retrieved from http://www.nhlbi.nih.gov/health/health-topics/topics/hdw.

10. Blankstein, R., Dr., Ward, R. P., Dr., Arnsdorf, M., Dr., Jones, B., Lou, Y., Dr., & Pine, M., Dr. (2005). "Female Gender Is an Independent Predictor of Operative Mortality After Coronary Artery Bypass Graft Surgery." Retrieved from http://circ.ahajournals.org/content/112/9_suppl/I-323.long.

11. "Heart Disease Facts." (2015, August 10). Retrieved from http://www.cdc.gov/heartdisease/facts.htm.

12. Framingham Heart Study. (n.d.). Retrieved from https://www.framinghamheartstudy.org/.

13. *Leisure Time Physical Activity of Moderate to Vigorous Intensity and Mortality: A Large Pooled Cohort Analysis* (2012). PLoS Med 9(11): e1001335. doi: 10.1371/journal.pmed.1001335.

14. "Adult Obesity Facts." (2015, September 21). Retrieved from http://www.cdc.gov/obesity/data/adult.html.

15. "Statistics About Diabetes." (2015, May 18). Retrieved from http://www.diabetes.org/diabetes-basics/statistics/.

16. "Heart attack symptoms." (n.d.). Retrieved from http://www.uptodate.com/contents/image?imageKey=PI/52579.

17. "Patent foramen ovale." *MedlinePlus Medical Encyclopedia.* (n.d.). Retrieved from https://www.nlm.nih.gov/medlineplus/ency/article/001113.htm.

18. Krasuski, R. A. (2010, August). "Congenital Heart Disease in the Adult." Retrieved from http://www.clevelandclinicmeded.com/medicalpubs/diseasemanagement/cardiology/congenital-heart-disease-in-the-adult/.

19. Jureidini, S. B., Appleton, R. S., Dr., Nouri, S., & Crawford, C. J. (1989, October). "Detection of coronary artery abnormalities in tetralogy of fallot by two-dimensional echocardiography." Retrieved from http://content.onlinejacc.org/article.aspx?articleid=1114007#tab1.

20. "Frequently Asked Questions." (2016, February 29). Retrieved from http://www.cdc.gov/alcohol/faqs.htm.

21. "HHS and USDA Release New Dietary Guidelines to Encourage Healthy Eating Patterns to Prevent Chronic Diseases." (2016, January). Retrieved from http://www.fns.usda.gov/pressrelease/2016/000516.

22. CY, C., & JY, C. (2009, December). "Essential fatty acids and human brain." Retrieved from http://www.ncbi.nlm.nih.gov/pubmed/20329590.

23. Reynolds, G. (2011, November 9). "Aging Well Through Exercise." Retrieved from http://well.blogs.nytimes.com/2011/11/09/aging-well-through-exercise/?utm_source=twitterfeed.

24. "Estimated Calorie Needs Per Day Table." (n.d.). Retrieved from http://www.cnpp.usda.gov/sites/default/files/usda_food_patterns/EstimatedCalorieNeedsPerDayTable.pdf.

25. "Eating Well As You Get Older." (2016, March). Retrieved from http://nihseniorhealth.gov/eatingwellasyougetolder/knowhowmuchtoeat/01.html.

26. US Department of Agriculture. (2010). *Dietary Guidelines for Americans, 2010.* Washington, DC: US Dept. of Health and Human Services, US Dept. of Agriculture.

27. "Chapter 2 Adequate Nutrients Within Calorie Needs." (2008, July 9). Retrieved from http://health.gov/dietaryguidelines/dga2005/document/html/chapter2.htm.

28. Robinson, J. (2013, May 25). "Breeding the Nutrition Out of Our Food." Retrieved from

http://www.nytimes.com/2013/05/26/opinion/sunday/bre
eding-the-nutrition-out-of-our-
food.html?pagewanted=all.

29. "Nutrition." (n.d.). Retrieved from
    http://www.cdhd.ne.gov/information/healthy-living-a-
    education/122-nutrition.
30. Vannice, G., & Rasmussen, H., Dr. (2014, January).
    "Position of the Academy of Nutrition and Dietetics:
    Dietary Fatty Acids for Healthy Adults." Retrieved from
    http://www.andjrnl.org/article/S2212-2672(13)01672-
    9/abstract.
31. "ACSM Issues New Recommendations on Quantity and
    Quality of Exercise." ACSM News Releases. American
    College of Sports Medicine. (Accessed 2016, May 27).
    Retrieved from http://www.acsm.org/about-acsm/media-
    room/news-releases/2011/08/01/acsm-issues-new-
    recommendations-on-quantity-and-quality-of-exercise.
32. "Exercise & Physical Activity: Your Everyday Guide
    from the National Institute on Aging." (2011, May).
    Retrieved from
    https://www.nia.nih.gov/health/publication/exercise-
    physical-activity/introduction.
33. Sink, K. M., Dr., Espeland, M. A., Dr., Castro, C. M., Dr.,
    & Church, T., Dr. (2015, August 25). "Effect of a 24-
    Month Physical Activity Intervention vs Health
    Education on Cognitive Outcomes in Sedentary Older
    Adults." Retrieved from
    http://jama.jamanetwork.com/article.aspx?articleid=24297
    12.
34. Currie L. Fall and Injury Prevention. In: Hughes RG,
    editor. *Patient Safety and Quality: An Evidence-Based
    Handbook for Nurses*. Rockville (MD): Agency for
    Healthcare Research and Quality (US); 2008 Apr. Chapter
    10. Available from
    http://www.ncbi.nlm.nih.gov/books/NBK2653/.

35. "Heart rate zones." Running for Fitness. (n.d.). Retrieved from http://www.runningforfitness.org/calc/heart-rate-calculators/hrzone.

36. Otto, M. W., & Smits, J. A. (2011). *Exercise for Mood and Anxiety: Proven Strategies for Overcoming Depression and Enhancing Well-Being.* New York, NY: Oxford University Press.

37. Strasser, B. (2012, November). "Physical activity in obesity and metabolic syndrome." Retrieved from http://www.ncbi.nlm.nih.gov/pmc/articles/PMC3715111/.

38. "ACSM Position Stand on Physical Activity and Weight Loss Now Available." (n.d.). Retrieved from https://www.acsm.org/about-acsm/media-room/acsm-in-the-news/2011/08/01/acsm-position-stand-on-physical-activity-and-weight-loss-now-available.

39. Plowman, S. A., & Smith, D. L. (2011). *Exercise Physiology for Health Fitness and Performance.* Philadelphia: Wolters Kluwer Health/Lippincott Williams & Wilkins.

40. "Unintentional Drowning: Get the Facts." (2014, April 28). Retrieved from http://www.cdc.gov/HomeandRecreationalSafety/Water-Safety/waterinjuries-factsheet.html.

41. "ABCs of a Safe Summer: Water Safety." (n.d.). Retrieved from http://www.redcross.org/images/MEDIA_CustomProductCatalog/m12140172_ABCs_of_Water_Safety.pdf.

42. "Drowning Risks in Natural Water Settings." (2012, June 13). Retrieved from http://www.cdc.gov/Features/dsDrowningRisks/.

43. "2015 National Livesaving Statistics." United States Lifesaving Association. (n.d.). Retrieved from http://arc.usla.org/Statistics/current.asp?Statistics=Current.

44. Dugdale, D. C., Dr., Zieve, D., Dr., & Black, B. (2013, May 2). "Nutrition and athletic performance." Retrieved from https://ufhealth.org/nutrition-and-athletic-performance.

45. Brosse, A. L., Sheets, E. S., Lett, H. S., & Blumenthal, J. A. (n.d.). "Exercise and the Treatment of Clinical Depression

in Adults." Retrieved from
http://web.colby.edu/essheets/files/2013/06/Exercise-and-
Clinical-Depression-Brosse-et-al.pdf.

46. "Life expectancy in the USA, 1900–98." (n.d.). Retrieved from
http://demog.berkeley.edu/~andrew/1918/figure2.html.

47. "Life Expectancy." (2015, January 20). Retrieved from
http://www.cdc.gov/nchs/fastats/life-expectancy.htm.

48. Martin Luther King, Jr. "I've Been to the Mountaintop."
(n.d.). Retrieved from
http://www.americanrhetoric.com/speeches/mlkivebeent
othemountaintop.htm.

49. Leal, A. C. (2013, January 28). "Why Does Your Skin
Age?" Retrieved from
http://dujs.dartmouth.edu/2013/01/why-does-your-skin-
age/#.VyjN5PmDFBd.

50. "Lung Capacity and Aging." (n.d.). Retrieved from
http://www.lung.org/lung-health-and-diseases/how-
lungs-work/lung-capacity-and-
aging.html?referrer=https://www.google.com/.

51. "An Age of Living Longer and Stronger." (2015, March
10). Retrieved from http://campusrec.unc.edu/2015/03/an-
age-of-living-longer-and-stronger/.

52. University of Michigan Health System. (2004, April 13).
"World's Oldest Mouse Reaches Milestone Birthday,
Teaches Scientists About Human Aging." *ScienceDaily*.
Retrieved May 3, 2016 from
www.sciencedaily.com/releases/2004/04/040412235951.htm.

53. Entringer, S., Epel, E. S., Lin, J., Buss, C., Shahbaba, B.,
Blackburn, E. H., . . . Wadhwa, P. D. (2014, February 1).
"Maternal psychosocial stress during pregnancy is
associated with newborn leukocyte telomere length."
Retrieved from
http://www.ncbi.nlm.nih.gov/pmc/articles/PMC3612534/.

ABOUT THE AUTHOR

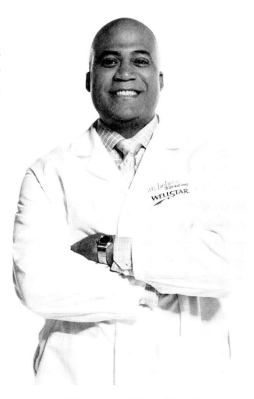

William A. Cooper is founding medical director of cardiovascular surgery at WellStar Health Systems in Marietta, Georgia, and former associate professor of surgery at Emory University in Atlanta, Georgia. He completed his BA/MD from the University of Missouri-Kansas City School of Medicine, post-graduate training in general surgery and cardiothoracic surgery at Emory University in Atlanta, Georgia, and his MBA from Emory University, Goizueta School of Business. Voted the 2015 Georgia Hospital Association Physician Hero, Dr. Cooper has served over thirty years in the United States Army Reserve and has completed three tours of duty in support of military operations around the world.